Additional praise for *Freedom from Pain*

"Pain is one of the most complex experiences in our existence and involves the physical, psychological, and spiritual dimensions of our life. *Freedom from Pain* approaches pain relief from all these dimensions in ways that have been clinically proven to work. Don't let pain dominate your life. Let Drs. Peter Levine and Maggie Phillips be your guides."

—LARRY DOSSEY, MD, author of *Healing Words*
and *The Power of Premonitions*

"Pain is unavoidable. Suffering is optional. Nice idea in principle, but how do we make it real? Peter and Maggie show you, step by step."

—SHINZEN YOUNG, author of *The Science of Enlightenment*

"With *Freedom from Pain,* the enigma of chronic, unrelenting pain seems much less mystifying. The gentle and reassuring approach of Drs. Levine and Phillips offers many practical possibilities for addressing pain with a sense of personal empowerment and a renewed drive toward wellness on *all* levels. Theirs is a multidimensional approach that holds great promise for providing the relief every person in pain hopes for."

—MICHAEL D. YAPKO, PHD, clinical psychologist and author of
Mindfulness and Hypnosis: The Power of Suggestion to Transform Experience and
Managing Pain With Hypnosis

Freedom

from

Pain

Freedom *from* Pain

DISCOVER YOUR
BODY'S POWER
TO OVERCOME
PHYSICAL PAIN

PETER A. LEVINE, PHD
MAGGIE PHILLIPS, PHD

sounds true
BOULDER, COLORADO

Sounds True, Inc.
Boulder, CO 80306

Copyright © 2012 Peter A. Levine and Maggie Phillips

Published 2012

Cover design by Jennifer Miles
Book design by Lisa Kerans

Printed in Canada

Library of Congress Cataloging-in-Publication Data

Levine, Peter A.
 Freedom from pain: discover your body's power to overcome physical pain
/ Peter A. Levine, Maggie Phillips.
    p. cm.
Includes biographical references and index.
ISBN 978-1-60407-663-9   *4966 9764 9/12*
1. Pain—Popular works. 2. Chronic pain—Popular works. 3. Mind and body
therapies—Popular works. I. Phillips, Maggie. II. Title.
RB127.L398 2012
616'.0472--dc23
                                    2011036499

ebook ISBN 978-1-60407-754-4

10   9 8 7 6 5 4 3 2 1

The pain is not to make you miserable,
the pain is to make you more aware!
And when you are aware, misery disappears.

—OSHO

The intensity of the pain depends on the degree
of resistance to the present moment,
and this in turn depends on how strongly you are
identified with your mind.

—ECKHART TOLLE

We are not victims of aging, sickness, pain and death.
These are part of scenery, not the seer,
who is immune to any form of change.
This seer is the spirit, the expression of eternal being.

—DEEPAK CHOPRA

Contents

Introduction

PAIN IS A POWERFUL WORD that triggers strong feelings—fear, anger, help-lessness, panic, and even grief. If you're one of the millions of people struggling with pain as you read this sentence, you are most certainly not alone. What mystifies patients, loved ones, and treating professionals alike is why pain persists long after an injury has healed, lingering for no apparent reason.

Like many others, you may have shuttled from doctor to doctor, diagnosis to diagnosis, and pain treatment to pain treatment. As your situation has become increasingly complex, you may have given up hope that your pain can shift and improve, and that you can become an authority over your pain, rather than your pain continuing to dominate you.

About two-thirds of the people in pain today have been living with significant pain for more than five years. In fact, the highest percentage of *all* medical visits is made to seek relief from pain. Yet this relief is often not easily found.

People with persistent and chronic pain struggle to find doctors who can effectively treat them. Untreated or undertreated pain is an ongoing epidemic. One recent study found that one out of four pain patients had changed doctors at least three times, citing the primary reason for change as that they still experienced significant pain. Other reasons given were that their pain was not taken seriously, that doctors were unwilling to treat their pain aggressively, and that doctors were without adequate knowledge to treat their pain effectively.[1]

A 2011 report issued by the Institute of Medicine (IOM) calls pain a "public health crisis," emphasizing that more people are suffering from chronic pain than from diabetes, cancer, and heart disease *combined*. The IOM study calls for better training in pain treatment at medical schools (since only five out of 133 medical schools surveyed currently require courses in pain management) and advocates continuing education training that helps keep professional knowledge current.[2]

A survey by the American Pain Society in 1999 indicated that more than 40 percent of the general population who suffered moderate to severe pain were unable to find adequate pain relief.[3] A report published in 2000 revealed that as many as 60 percent of the respondents believed that pain is just something you have to live with, and 28 percent felt there was no solution to their pain.[4]

Pain has an enormous impact on quality of life at any age, constricting the ability to work, socialize, exercise, concentrate, perform simple tasks, and sleep. Yet even though there are ever-increasing numbers of new methods being created to resolve and relieve pain, there appears to be an even greater surge of pain conditions with new names, causes, theories, and drugs to treat them.

The cost of unmanaged suffering is huge. Part of the reason for this problem is that pain is so complex—ranging far beyond the intersection of neural transmission and sensory experience. The puzzle of pain involves a complicated labyrinth of emotions, sensations, culture, individual experience, genetics, spiritual meaning, as well as habitual physiological reactions, and some experts believe that chronic pain for many patients has become a disease in itself.[5]

Because pain is such a complex puzzle, no single health care perspective or discipline holds the particular puzzle piece that brings a universal solution. Never before has there been such a vast array of therapeutic options for pain, ranging from Western medicine to traditional Chinese medicine approaches such as acupuncture and acupressure; chiropractic, nutritional, and supplemental care; hypnosis, special types of imagery (including guided imagery), and other psychological methods; and bodywork, yoga, and massage, just to name a few.

What does this mean for the pain patient? Frequently, individuals in pain are thrown into increasing confusion in their relentless search for tools that will ultimately bring an end to their suffering. Yet the real power of most pain-treatment methods to bring lasting results lies not within the methods, but in their unique application in alignment with each individual's needs, beliefs, personality, and experience. While each method is promising in what it can offer, the key puzzle piece remains *your* contribution—the responses *you* bring to your own healing process.

There is every reason to believe that the unique qualities of each individual impact and shape painful experience and also provide the platform for resilience and recovery. From our perspective, the one ingredient of individual experience that has not been sufficiently considered in usual attempts to solve the puzzle of pain is *the role of unresolved trauma* that is held in the body. For example, we know that a high percentage of all chronic pain patients also struggle with some form of traumatic stress. Research has shown that chronic pain may not only be caused by physical injury, but also by stress and emotional issues. In fact, people who suffer from PTSD (post-traumatic stress disorder) are at a much higher risk for developing chronic pain.[6]

The presence of unreleased traumatic experience changes everything when it comes to the treatment of pain. Both of us have found consistently, in our collective clinical experience spanning more than eighty years, that whenever we have worked with pain that does not respond to usual treatments, the reason inevitably lies in what accumulated stress and trauma contribute to the pain picture. In this program, we distill the best of our thinking and practices to empower you to identify and master the patterns of stress that create and contribute to pain. We will sometimes use examples from our clinical practice to illustrate things that you can do to help resolve your pain. Indeed, we also strongly suggest professional help, when it would be of benefit to you.

We frequently work with people who suffer from neck, back, and shoulder pain related to motor vehicle accidents. Many of them come to us because they are not responding to usual prescriptions of medication, physical therapy, and other treatment approaches. When we explore further, we often find that what blocks their progress is the residue of previous accidents or injuries that seem unrelated to the current one that has triggered their pain. Once we help them to unwind the nervous system responses to accumulated stresses from multiple incidents that may have created traumatic stress, they begin to recover quickly and completely.

We have found it important to address trauma at several different levels:

- **Working with trauma that may have caused the pain through accident, injury, disease, or other overwhelming events.** Usually these are thought of as the *precipitating* events or triggers. Although it is not necessary to relive overwhelming or painful events that are contributing to your pain, it is important to explore how the event has created or contributed to specific patterns of distress and dysregulation or lack of balance. The good news is that you will be learning simple ways to help you regulate or shift the way your body feels, so that balance and comfort return naturally and reliably.

- **Discovering how persistent emotional and physical pain become traumatizing.** If you weren't depressed or anxious before your injury or accident or whatever caused your pain condition, the pain itself is a significant stressor that can create those reactions. These traumatic reactions can be strong enough for

individuals in pain who have a strong trauma history
to receive a diagnosis of PTSD.

- **Identifying unresolved trauma predating the
pain condition that gets stirred up by the current
pain problem.** For example, traumatizing illness,
hospitalizations, and surgeries under the age of five
can set the stage for later panic attacks and excess pain
related to even a routine dental surgery later in adult life.

- **Exploring early childhood trauma, such as birth,
perinatal, postnatal stress, and attachment trauma,
which becomes a barrier to trusting the body and
other people to help.** We commonly find that people
in unrelenting pain did not learn early in life how
to regulate uncomfortable or distressing experiences.
Frequently, this is because they did not have help
and support in doing so when they were too young
to regulate themselves. They may have been either
neglected or hurt if they expressed distress. If you
have difficulty in this area, you may not have had
experiences of early comfort that you could learn to
internalize and apply as effective soothing and self-
regulation skills when your pain developed. You will
learn some of these important regulation skills during
the *Freedom from Pain* program.

Although doctors commonly use the word "trauma" in describing some
sources of pain, they rarely understand how important treating the
effects of trauma can be in resolving pain, nor do they know how to go
about this. While an important goal in our practice is to train professionals to identify and treat the interactions of pain and trauma, the

message of this particular program is that there are simple practices that *anyone* in pain can learn and use. These practices can reverse pain and bring lasting relief from endless suffering through the gentle release of trauma reactions that have been held in the body.

Many people ask us, "Why do I still have such intense pain even though my doctors tell me that the physical causes of my pain have healed and I've explored all of the treatment methods that any professional has recommended to me? Why do I still hurt?" This program will provide answers to this compelling question, so that your pain is no longer so mysterious to you. We will also teach you simple strategies that you can learn to use effectively in order to recruit your body as your main ally in obtaining lasting freedom from both pain and suffering.

Three essential principles frame what we believe and teach, and form the context of our approach:

1. No one can heal effectively and efficiently from emotional, physical, or spiritual pain and suffering without involving the body at the center of their healing process. This has, of course, been Peter's life work and the foundation for his Somatic Experiencing® (SE) model. This truth has also been, in a different way, the root of Maggie's essential beliefs about healing, a thread which she has interwoven through Somatic Experiencing practice into other disciplines, including EMDR (eye movement desensitization and reprocessing), hypnosis, ego-state therapy, and energy psychology approaches.

   Somatic Experiencing (www.traumahealing.com) is a naturalistic, body-awareness approach to the healing of trauma being taught throughout the world. It is the result of over forty years of observation, research, and hands-on development by Peter and his students.

Based upon the realization that human beings have an innate ability to overcome the effects of stress and trauma, Somatic Experiencing restores self-regulation and returns a sense of aliveness, resilience, and wholeness to traumatized individuals who have had these precious gifts taken away. This work has been applied to combat veterans; rape survivors; Holocaust survivors; auto accident, post-surgical trauma, and chronic pain sufferers; and even to infants who have suffered traumatic births.

The Freedom from Pain program will teach you step-by-step how to reconnect with your body's resources in ways that will not only comfort and relieve your pain, but also provide an ultimate solution to what has caused and continues to maintain your suffering. Some of the tools we teach may work dramatically for you, and others may have little effect or are not appropriate in terms of timing. We encourage you to take what helps (even a little) and leave what doesn't. Most importantly, we will teach you how your body can be your most valuable ally in your healing process instead of the painful enemy that relentlessly blocks your forward progress.

2. We acknowledge, due to the inherent complexity of pain, that no one method works for everyone. What works best is a toolbox of methods that you can apply to achieve reliable relief and ultimate freedom from the tyranny of pain in your life. An important predictor of your success is *you*—your willingness to experiment until you determine what really does help with your pain.

One of the many challenges to holding a flexible focus is the fact that pain is so dynamic, changing unexpectedly in form and location. As your pain shifts and changes in response to the tools you learn, your need to modify those tools will change too. So in addition to persistence and trust, we encourage you to practice openness of mind, heart, and spirit so that you can learn how to befriend the natural resources of your body.

3. The tools you will learn from us are only the beginning. How you learn to use them to achieve creative and successful self-regulation is what will create movement and momentum toward expansion, resilience, and flow, and reverse the vicious cycle of pain, fear, and suffering.

Self-regulation is the cornerstone of our approach in *Freedom from Pain*. In general, learning to regulate the emotional and physical states that may be linked to your suffering is what will bring you into a collaborative alliance between mind, emotion, and spiritual awareness, through body experience. The moment-to-moment ability to regulate your most painful emotions and body sensations will also create a healthy balance between independence and the ability to find help in your connections with others.

HOW TO USE THIS PROGRAM

In order to help you navigate your journey through this program, we have organized the book as follows:

Chapter 1 is a general overview of how we hurt and why we suffer. We suggest some first steps for body exploration and an exercise to teach you to reinhabit your body.

Chapter 2 shows how people in pain can get stuck in the
pain trap and includes two foundational exercises to
help you move out of the trap toward freedom.

Chapter 3 explains how we shift from normal, necessary pain
to chronic pain. This chapter includes a wide range of
tools and exercises for beginning to intervene in chronic
pain. Specifically, it offers strategies for dealing effectively
with dissociation; anxiety, fear, and panic; helplessness
and hopelessness; and anger, rage, and irritability.

Chapter 4 explores the first two stages in the three-
stage journey back from pain: stage one, achieving
reliable self-regulation; and stage two, ongoing
transformation. This chapter includes five exercises.

Chapter 5 provides information on working with specific
pain conditions and syndromes. We recommend
you read about these, even if you do not suffer from
the designated problem, since each discussion offers
valuable insight into working with all types of pain.

Chapter 6 concerns preventing and resolving the pain
of medical trauma. This chapter includes advice on
creating a pain plan for upcoming medical procedures.

Chapter 7 discusses the third stage of the journey back from
pain into resilience, continued recovery, and restoration
of the deep self. It is designed to help you set your course
for further growth and the development of a life that
is truly free from pain and infused with vitality and
forward direction.

We have also included specific examples from our clients so that you can see how this program has worked with a wide variety of people and pain issues. Please note that although the stories are true, we do not use the patients' real names in order to protect their privacy.

HOW TO USE THE PRACTICE EXERCISES

The backbone of this program is composed of audio practice exercises. You will find them on the audio CD that accompanies this book. The audio program offers a different opportunity to interact with the material we have included. We recognize that some people like to work with the written word, some with audio, and many with a combination of the two. We have tried to provide multiple options so you can see what works best for you. The important thing is to feel free to experiment, rather than trying to make any one component of the program exclusive.

We have included fifteen exercises in the audio program. Whenever an exercise has a corresponding audio track, we will note this under the exercise heading so it's easy for you to find. You will notice that although the audio exercises follow the same outline as the written exercises, they are slightly different. The beauty of the audio format is that it gives us the opportunity to expand the exercises a bit, and therefore offer you yet another way of working with this material.

We recommend that when listening to the audio exercises, you create an environment that will support a productive focus. This might include eliminating background noises by turning off your cell phone, for instance, wearing comfortable clothes, and placing yourself in a position that supports your body fully. Please, never listen to the audio exercises while driving.

We have also included a number of "mini exercises" within the written program. These are opportunities to practice applying some of the principles we present "in the moment" in relation to your body experiences. In order to maximize your success with the audio as well as written practice exercises, we also encourage you to create a pain journal.

HOW TO USE A PAIN JOURNAL

We have had many experiences in helping clients keep and maintain a pain notebook or journal as part of their work with us. You may have been assigned this task at some point, or have chosen on your own to begin journaling as part of moving forward with your growth in some way. Hopefully, you have found this to be helpful in the past, or perhaps you have not persisted long enough or in a way that allowed you to experience success.

Over the years, we have discussed with our clients what has been helpful for them in reaching success with many types of pain. Many of them have mentioned that keeping a pain diary or journal was specifically related to achieving freedom from pain. As an example, Julie, who had struggled with chronic pelvic pain due to endometriosis and scar tissue from several related surgeries, commented at her last session, "I know I resisted keeping a journal. But it wasn't until you gave me specific assignments for how and when to track my pain that I began to build positive momentum. Before that, I wasn't really dealing with what was actually happening, but instead with what I wished were true or was afraid was true about my pain."

Although we suggest that you track your progress with practice exercises throughout our program, we hope that you will expand beyond keeping notes about your practice results. It's also important to practice rating your pain on a 0–10 pain scale at least once a day (0=no pain and 10=unbearable pain) and to log the types of sensations you are experiencing. If you are not experiencing forward progress with your pain, you may need to "take your pain temperature" three to four times per day so that you get a more complete and accurate picture of your patterns with pain.[7]

For additional results, you may also find it helpful to chart sudden increases in pain and note any triggers that may have influenced those, as well as noting interventions, activities, and experiences that preceded low pain ratings. It can also be useful to chart the times you take medications and supplements, recording any positive results you are observing as well as negative side effects.

Journaling is an excellent way to keep track of your progress through the *Freedom from Pain* program and to help you learn to track your pain sensations more effectively. We also include one audio journaling practice exercise (see track 14) to encourage the development of this important skill. Look for this journal icon at the end of each written exercise to remind you to use your pain journal.

We are grateful that you are entrusting us with this opportunity to teach you what we have learned from many people like you about full recovery from the trauma of pain. We hope that what you learn and practice with us will guide you to reclaim your wholeness and bring you the peace that makes life fully worth living.

CHAPTER ONE

Why We Hurt and How We Suffer

It is life's only true opponent.
Only Fear can defeat life.
—*LIFE OF PI*, YAN MARTEL

THOSE OF US FORTUNATE ENOUGH to engage in a life fully lived will find it nearly impossible to escape from this world without experiencing moments of significant pain. According to the Buddha, "When touched with a feeling of pain, the ordinary person laments . . . becomes distraught . . . *contracts* and so . . . feels two pains . . . just as if they were to shoot a man with an arrow and, right afterward, were to shoot him with another so that he would feel the pain of [both] . . ."

The first arrow in this teaching represents necessary pain. The second one represents unnecessary suffering and trauma. It is our *fear about pain* that creates this second arrow, a fear that creates a fertile landscape for chronic pain, distress, and anguish. As pain sufferers, we become so frightened of pain that we recoil from feeling *any* bodily sensations. It is as though we believe that by feeling our bodies we will

1

be destroyed or, at the very least, our conditions will worsen. Hence we remain stuck and so shoot ourselves with the second arrow.

In this volume, we hope to provide you with the skills necessary to begin to help take the fear and hurt out of your pain. This program provides you with the means to *prevent* chronic pain from developing in the aftermath of *common* life events such as accidents and surgeries, as well as to release unresolved pain that has been held in the body from past traumatic events.

It is our shared vision that, with the guidance of this program, you will start to free yourselves from unnecessary suffering. Our wish is to support your transformation of pain into an empowering energy that allows you to embrace your life fully, with purpose, and with freedom from pain.

If you are reading this book, we're imagining that you've been struggling with pain or that you care about someone who is. More than likely, you have in mind important questions and concerns that you want to make sure are addressed in this program.

We want to assure you right from the beginning that our purpose is to introduce you to practical, effective strategies distilled from working successfully with many different pain problems over the years. Practice exercises sprinkled throughout our program, beginning with this first chapter, will help you understand the main principles and further evolve related techniques into integrated skills.

Some of the important questions we will answer include:

- What does the latest research teach us about how to resolve pain and suffering?
- How do I prioritize my many needs so that I stop feeling overwhelmed and can begin to reduce my pain right away?
- Will this approach work with *my* specific type of pain?
- How can I get the support I need from professionals who work with me, as well as from my loved ones?

- How can I make decisions about medical
  interventions including medication and surgery?

We'll begin now with a foundational question—what *is* pain, anyway?

WHAT IS PAIN?

Pain, first and foremost, is a signal to let us know that we have been injured or are ill. Pain can also arise from tension and discomfort caused by how we respond to stress and threat. When we are threatened physically, emotionally, mentally, and spiritually, our nervous systems automatically react to ensure that we are protected from harm or injury.

In its purest form, pain is an essential part of our natural survival system, warning us that something is wrong and motivating us to give our body urgent attention. Pain signals are sent from nerves in the part of the body that has been injured to the brain. No pain is felt until the brain has interpreted the information it has received.

Many parts of the brain, as we shall see, collaborate in turning on pain as a survival response, including areas that govern past memories, emotions, and mood, as well as future intentions. Meaning and importance of the pain are also part of the pain picture. For instance, the same hand injury might mean something very different to a professional pianist than it does to an amateur volleyball player; therefore, both individuals may have drastically different pain experiences. That is why each person's struggle with pain will be unique, and why we actively encourage you to find the exercises and concepts in this program that work best for you.

We will be studying three types of pain in this program: physical, emotional, and posttraumatic. Physical pain is due to actual injury and tissue damage. Emotionally based pain is formed by strong, unresolved emotions that we have "stored" in the body instead of healthfully expressing them. Finally, posttraumatic pain is generated from much stronger reactions to overwhelming, terrifying, or devastating events.

These three types of pain are categorized according to their root causes, which also often correspond to how they appear or present themselves. For example, following an accident or injury, your primary concern will almost always be the localized physical pain you experience. When you suffer the loss of someone you love, as expected, you will struggle with emotional distress that might include sadness, grief, fear, anger, rage, despair, or some combination of these feelings. And, after being assaulted, threatened with rape, or surviving a fire, flood, or tornado that results in the loss of all your belongings and perhaps even family members, you more than likely will be overwhelmed by posttraumatic reactions that might include insomnia, panic attacks, sensory flashbacks, or systemic or stress-related pain such as migraines, depression, helplessness, and hopelessness.

Although these three classifications have obvious distinctions, one of the keys to treating pain successfully is the recognition that these three basic types overlap each other. Pain then is multi-dimensional. For example, many physical pain conditions include emotional reactions and interactions with past trauma. Most emotional pain conditions will also feature somatic symptoms such as physical pain and links to past traumatic events. And posttraumatic conditions involve a complex combination of all three types of pain responses.

So in addition to presenting ways to help you achieve freedom from these three types of pain, we will also help you understand some of the complexity that may be driving *your* pain and preventing you from healing. Because most pain complexity is linked to trauma, we continue our opening discussion with important perspectives on trauma.

WHAT IS TRAUMA?

There are many theories about what trauma is. However, most definitions emphasize that the traumatized person has been exposed to one or more life events involving actual (or perceived) threats to survival or physical wholeness, and where the individual's reactions included intense negative emotions like fear, helplessness, loss of control, and/ or terror. Traumatic events are basically of two types—a single incident (such as an accident or injury), or multiple, ongoing events like those involved in repeated childhood emotional, physical, or sexual abuse, and/or neglect.

Studies of animal responses to threat have helped us better understand how these kinds of responses are resolved and released. Animals in the wild encounter numerous incidents of threat to their survival each day, yet generally seem to display no residual signs of trauma. From what we know, animals in their wild habitats are only concerned with what is happening *right now*. They do not worry or dream about the future. They do not regret or pine for the past. They are always "in the moment," so to speak. After the threat has passed, they give themselves time to "discharge" or release the energy generated by the threat, and allow themselves time to settle. This is what we will be teaching you to do in this program: to become aware of your heightened physiological responses, to learn and practice a variety of techniques to discharge energies related to high-threat arousal, and strategies to give yourself time to settle from this activation and return to equilibrium.

The main difference between wild animals and human ones in terms of trauma is that animals *complete* fight and flight responses that allow them to fight back against what threatens them or to flee and escape the source of threat. Then they spontaneously shake off any residual stress effects through a series of shaking movements. It is after these involuntary trembling movements reach their natural conclusion that animals are able to become fully mobile and return to life as usual. They are also freed from the aftereffects of traumatic stress.

We human animals, however, often cannot escape or fight back, and have been conditioned not to allow our bodies time to "shake off" the aftermath of threat. We then often shift into the freeze response. Remnants of the fight, flight, or freeze response, when not released from the body, leave us in these heightened and inhibited physiological states. In order to try to integrate back into society (where we often receive the message to "just get over it"), we try to suppress these urges to fight back or flee. This avoidance can create more physiological constriction and psychological dissociation, the foundation for many pain conditions.

During this program, you will learn more about the somatic reactions that set the stage for the evolution of stress and pain disorders as well as ways to free your body of their effects. The unique contribution of the Somatic Experiencing model to the treatment of pain and trauma is the understanding that trauma exists in the nervous system and the body, not in the content of the traumatizing event.

The Freedom from Pain process emphasizes "bottom-up" approaches, or healing from the body level up to intervene in related thoughts, feelings, and perceptions. To accomplish this, you will learn a series of skills related to first identifying and then regulating your pain sensations. This will allow you to gradually break free of the pain trap that may be blocking your recovery (see page 19), and eventually release the intense energies trapped in the nervous system so that they can be transformed into resilience and flow.

THE LANGUAGE OF SENSATION

In order to recruit your body as your ally in securing freedom from pain, the first step is to learn how to communicate with your body so that you can create a healing, collaborative partnership. In other words, you will need to figure out how to shift your body from painful enemy to invaluable resource.

Although it's obvious that the body is important to the healing process, many people in pain have trained themselves to disconnect from their body experience in a defensive attempt to avoid feeling more pain. Yet leaving body experience out of your healing equation will greatly limit your healing possibilities.

During this program, we will teach you to develop the *language of sensation* so that you can recognize the wisdom of your body in terms of the important information and feedback it provides. The *felt sense* paradigm of Focusing, developed by philosopher, psychologist, and researcher Eugene Gendlin, provides a map for learning this new language.[1]

The felt sense utilizes the language of body-mind communication and serves as a kind of radar or navigation system, letting us know instantly about elements of our internal and external environments and how they are affecting us in the current moment. Understandings from Somatic Experiencing and our Freedom from Pain program will prepare you to listen to and interpret this language as guidance, relayed to you immediately through your felt-sense radar.

You can learn, step-by-step, to decode the power of the unspoken voice of the sensate communications your body transmits. This will enable you to follow your body's primitive, nonverbal pathways to discover actions that you can take to release the shock of trauma and pain. Tracking these kinds of sensory, nonverbal clues can also lead you to resources of expansion that can relieve your suffering and help reset your nervous system to support balance and new awareness.

First Steps

As part of your Freedom from Pain program, we recommend, if you aren't already, engaging in gentle movement, such as stretching, qi gong, tai chi, or a gentle, restorative yoga class for people with injuries or disabilities.

Receiving gentle massage can also be helpful.[2] As you explore your body experience with the help of an experienced masseuse, you can begin to realize numerous important pain connections. For example, you may recognize that the pain in your shoulder or neck may actually start down in your hips and back. The pain in your back could also originate from constriction in your ankles and knees. Massage can help you relax and also become aware of how various types of tension in your body create the pain.

In movement classes, you can practice the same principles, by moving slowly, and beginning to become aware of the tense muscles in the center of your body, and then the muscles at the periphery. Also note any images or feelings that you may have as you slowly allow yourself to release the tension through the gentle movements you are experiencing.

Our caveat is that massage and movement practice should never be painful (or that the pain should dissipate quickly and you should feel less pain afterwards). You must take care never to let your massage or movement practices become so intense that you have to ignore or push through the pain.

The first stepping stones on this journey are often ones of *invitation* and *permission* for simple exploration, using little more than innate curiosity and focused attention. This first exercise will help you begin to reconnect with and re-inhabit your body, which you may have abandoned to the ravages of pain and trauma. Although this may sound like a major undertaking, our message is that there are simple practices that can help you befriend your body and its unique resources.

EXERCISE: Re-Inhabiting Your Body
◀)) Track 1

Let's start with a part of your body that is not painful. It's important to note that no matter how long you have been in pain, there is always a place in your body that is relatively pain-free. Granted, this part of your body may be small and off the beaten path, so to speak, like the inside of your forearm or the palm of your hand. Wherever it is, find and feel the lack of pain, the pleasure or comfort, or at least the neutrality of sensation.

Now allow yourself to feel an area where your body hurts. Take this at your own pace, and if it's too intense, find an area that is less painful, and one that you can stay with more comfortably. Gently sense the contours of this area by breathing into it, and then see if you can let go of pain or tension as you exhale. Some of the sensations you may find are tingling, burning, warmth or heat, coldness, sharpness, stabbing, or aching.[3] Whatever sensations you discover, just notice how they change with your awareness and breath.

Next, return to the pain-free area you identified before, sensing into it as you breathe in, and then letting go of what you sense there as you breathe out. Repeat this several times. What are you finding now in this area of the body that you did not find before?

Using your breath, shift back and forth, visiting several of the more painful places in your body, and then the more pleasant or pain-free places. Pause at each, sending your breath to re-inhabit it, and letting go of all effort as you exhale.

Record your responses to this exercise in your pain notebook.

BILL: BEGINNING THE SENSATE JOURNEY

Bill discovered the tools of invitation and permission in his first consultation session, which he had scheduled to evaluate the persistent nerve pain just below his right scapula following a serious bicycle accident.

Bill was pacing, his face guarded as he waited to find out how this appointment would be different from the numerous sessions with the acupuncturists, physiatrists, orthopedists, osteopaths, physical therapists, kinesiologists, surgeons, and medical doctors he had already experienced during the seven years following his bicycle accident.

Describing the site of the pain, he commented, "It's hard for me to believe I still have this. No one can find a reason for this pain." As with so many pain sufferers, nothing had shown up on any of the X-rays, CAT scans, and MRIs. The only finding had resulted from a nerve conduction test indicating that an auxiliary nerve had been compressed. "But I'll tell you," he added, "it's very real to me. I feel like I died that day I went off my bike. I don't remember it, but I know it happened, and in that moment, everything in my life changed."

With some reassurance and encouragement, Bill told the story he had told countless times before. Instead of passively accepting his narration—which is what Bill had experienced in all his previous medical visits—I began to probe for the impact that the story was having on Bill's body, and, at the same time, initiating the process of resolution.

Bill explained that at the time of his accident, he had been trying out a new racing bike. Hunched over the handlebars, head down, Bill failed to see a telephone repair truck parked in the bike lane (later he found out that there was no orange cone marking its presence), sailed over the handlebars, and crashed headfirst into the left side of the truck's bumper. Twelve hours later, he woke up in the hospital with no memory of what had happened. After his release, the officers who had been called to the scene told Bill and his family that he had answered all of their questions accurately with the exception of giving them an inaccurate phone number.

When I asked Bill to show me how he believed the impact occurred, Bill got up from his chair and began making movements related to losing control of the bicycle. Knowing that, to be effective, any movements needed to go very slowly to aid in regulation and integration, I suggested that he continue the movements as if in "slow motion."

After several sequences of movement, Bill commented, "That's interesting. This is the first time I've realized how I must have landed on my right shoulder. I didn't hit on the top of my shoulder, as I've been thinking all this time. It has to be that my body twisted to the left to try to avoid hitting the truck, so that's why the force of the impact was really right under my scapula where the pain still is."

Because Bill was helped to connect with his felt sense of what had happened, allowing his body to take the lead, he was able to regain a valuable clue about the site of his pain. Instead of the scapula pain being an indirect, mysterious result of his collision with the truck, he discovered that the area of chronic, lingering pain was likely one of the epicenters of the impact. This connection helped him to make sense of his body's story.

We also spent time exploring other accidents and injuries seemingly unrelated to the injuries from his bike accident. Bill's initial response to this inquiry was: "I've never really hurt my shoulder before." However, after a series of probing questions about surgery, accidents, and injuries, Bill realized he had had several related accidents. These included an earlier head injury sustained during his short history as a high school football player, a bad fall where his right hip and right upper body landed on a set of concrete steps, as well as an even earlier accident in first grade when he fell down a flight of steps and landed on his left hip.

The second clue Bill discovered in his history was the presence of shock and dissociation that protected him from immediate pain after both hip injuries. After both of those falls, Bill reported that he had continued activity as if nothing had happened, until finally others suggested he get medical attention. X-rays revealed that his left hip had been cracked by the fall in first grade, and that his body later was misaligned in his cervical spine and pelvis. During the second fall on his right hip, the same side of his body as the bike collision, he felt "stunned," but got up and continued to play ball, though he sought medical attention later.

This ability to "push through the pain" was echoed in his revelations of two other severe accidents sustained as a young man. In the first of these, he and his (now) wife had just announced their engagement to her parents and they were all enjoying time on the family boat when it was hit from behind by a bigger boat, slamming all four adults into the water. Bill reported that his right arm was "frozen" holding his fiancé tight to protect her from harm from the time they hit the water until rescue.

As soon as they fell in the water, he felt something moving across his back from right to left, and immediately recognized that it was the side of the other boat that had hit them. He recalled, "All I could think was that I had to push us away from the propeller. So I was holding on to Millie with my right arm and pushing away as hard as I could with my left leg and my left arm." As he swiveled to show me what had happened, he noticed that his body had attempted to brace to protect his fiancé on his right side while bracing against the threat of the boat and its propeller on his left side.

When I asked what it was like for him to feel those movements, Bill said, "I realize now that the other boat went right across the area where my scapula pain is from my bike accident. Do you think the two accidents are connected somehow?" He also recognized that his body was divided between holding on to Millie, who was clutching her engagement ring, and desperately trying to flee from the boat's invasion on the other side.

Bill's story illustrates the fact that although he was not practiced in connecting with his body experience, with guidance he discovered during his first sensate journey several important links between traumatic events and his current physical pain. He also began to realize that some of the movements his body made to protect him had also played an important part in his pain story. These discoveries activated his curiosity, which helped him to begin trusting the wisdom of his body and continued to be an invaluable tool in resolving his pain. In later sessions, learning to use the language of sensation allowed him to feel more deeply the connections between the various somatic responses to these traumatic events, and to begin to shift the pain itself in a positive direction.

Bill's story is also a good example of the fusion of the three types of pain we mentioned earlier (see page 3). In addition to the physical scapula pain and the posttraumatic pain related to the series of earlier injuries and the boating accident, Bill later realized that unconscious emotional feelings of fear and loss contributed to his pain reactions as well as to his challenges in resolving them.

THE THREAT RESPONSE AND PAIN

An important aspect of trauma is the threat response. The threat of danger mobilizes our call to action, an all-hands-on-deck response, and turns on the classic fight-or-flight system that we have mentioned before, and which you are probably familiar with. Certain nervous-system networks (the sympathetic adrenal system, in particular) are engaged to prepare vital organs and muscles for these protective responses. Like little batteries, our nerve cells charge up so they can fire off commands to the body to preserve life, whether it is for that extra burst of speed or one more good punch.

When the threat is perceived potentially fatal or as inescapable, the third natural response to threat, the freeze response, is evoked. Here, we lie immobile waiting for the threat to pass. This collapse response is often referred to as dissociation. When we become stuck in this state, we feel frozen in life, unable to move forward.

Our protective responses would be ideal in situations where we can actively defend ourselves. When fight-or-flight responses are impossible—when the animal (human or otherwise) cannot fight back against the threat or escape it—then like turtles, our heads retract into our shoulders and we bring our shoulders up toward our ears. Our bodies, particularly our musculoskeletal systems, tighten and brace. We may freeze in a kind of paralysis or collapse into helplessness, despair, and dissociation.

It may seem odd that dissociating or disconnecting from the body can become part of a pain problem. Dissociation, however, doesn't turn off the fear or pain but protectively walls it off so we don't feel it. This diminishes our capacity to feel pleasure and to think clearly. Dissociation prevents us from being in the here-and-now.

Frank had had more than twenty surgical procedures on his knee, including three full knee replacements. For most of the procedures and surgeries, he was dissociated from his body and so had manageable pain afterwards. When he approached the final surgery that ultimately brought him to treatment, however, he was scared for the first time, scared of the pain and scared of what the effects of the procedure would be.

When he woke up from this surgery in the hospital, he was in excruciating pain and asked for more medication. When the nurse explained that the doctor had not left orders for more medication than she had given him, Frank announced that if she did not find a way to give him the medication, he would tear apart the ICU. When Frank's dissociative barrier was breached, he was overcome with terror and by the terrible pain that had been managed by the walls of dissociation his nervous system had constructed. As he began to feel these feelings again, his brain turned on the fight response to protect him from these perceived threats.

Another issue is that many different situations can activate the threat response. Some situations, like assault, actually are life threatening, yet others are based more on our perceptions that something *appears* to be life threatening. For example, the boss at work may be unsatisfied with an employee's work on a project. The employee may be called into the office for a meeting. Suddenly, a spike in the employee's heart rate and respiration may signal preparation for life-saving action because of the *perception* that if the job is in jeopardy, the employee's chances of survival are lost too. Therefore, the situation is perceived as a threat to life itself rather than just a situation that needs to be attended to.

In other cases, such as the dangerous threat of an automobile accident, since there is no human or animal to fight back against or to flee from, the fight and flight reactions become internal ones. These protective reactions not only are dysfunctional, they become habitual and can contribute to many health problems, including pain.

CHARGE, DISCHARGE, SETTLE

As mentioned previously, if the roots of our responses to threat are directly related to the pain we experience, then we can learn a lot about how to complete these survival responses and release the energy engendered by threat by studying animals in the wild. This is because animals in their natural habitats don't become traumatized in the same ways, or as easily, as people, pets, or animals in captivity.

Imagine a rabbit in a small glen, munching on some green grass. A sound comes from the bushes. The rabbit's ears, followed by its head, perk up and turn toward the sound to locate its source and whether it is a threat to life. From out of the foliage, a coyote sprints into view. The chase is on: the rabbit's muscles engage and dig into the ground as it sets off, hoping to escape through several daring twists and turns. Ultimately the rabbit uses its resources of speed and agility (and a bit of good luck) to escape and then hides in a log or down inside a hole. Finally safe, the rabbit takes a series of deep breaths and shakes off its encounter with threat.

Rabbits, like most other animals, are equipped to utilize flight, fight, or freeze responses to survive the threats they encounter. So the wild animal that may encounter these types of life-threatening situations multiple times a day must be equipped so that it doesn't carry residual stress. Otherwise, it would lose its capacity to fight back or flee.

The question is: what's the difference between the reactions of a human being and those of an animal in terms of trauma? This is an important concern, because if an animal became traumatized as readily as a human being, the animal and its entire species might not survive. In fact, precisely because it can release the stress of threat and learn new escape moves, the animal may actually become more effective in evading threat each time it's challenged.

After a threatening encounter, as mentioned earlier in this chapter, animal bodies tend to shake and tremble for a relatively short period as part of moving out of a shock reaction. This is illustrated in the behavior of the opossum. If attacked by a predator, the opossum freezes, or "plays possum." This is not "playing," but is actually a response to threat defined by a profound physiological shut down: this is often its only option since the opossum can't run away because it's very slow, and is unable to fight back because it lacks sharp teeth and claws.

After the threat passes, however, the opossum doesn't immediately jump up and run away and go about the business of hunting for grubs or engaging in a complex mating ritual. After several minutes (or up to several hours), the opossum slowly begins to move, though it's still unstable. It shakes and trembles a little bit, and then seems to regain its grounding, and off it goes. Animals that are slow or unequipped relative to their predators often default automatically into this freeze or immobility strategy. This is often times the case with humans, particularly children. For example, if children who are abused try to fight back, this will often make the situation worse. The only option that children have is to collapse, which is why they're so vulnerable to trauma, particularly when they are not guided toward recovery time, and encouraged to shake and tremble, and to finally fall back into a deep settling in themselves and their environment.

The innate biological responses of animals help them literally shake off the result of their traumatic encounters and then they automatically return to equilibrium, since equilibrium and balance are the patterns most established in nature. Animals go on to another experience or a new day. Because humans frequently block these recovery reactions, this benefit of shaking off the impact of threat and trauma may escape us. That is, until we are guided to recover the wisdom of nature.

HOMEOSTASIS AND THE RHYTHMS OF LIFE

Our program will teach you to learn to identify and accept, or at least not interfere with, your own innate healing responses so that you can move into truer alignment with your hard-wired animal heritage. This type of learning will teach you to become curious about and then begin to explore the dynamics that underlie your pain and help restore your animal nature.

Much of this program is designed to teach you how to discover and befriend the body sensations that are connected to trauma and, more importantly, with resilience. We've found that acceptance of the full range of those somatic responses is what prompts the nervous system to restore balance automatically.

To practice this kind of awareness at this moment, read aloud the words "fear," "anger," "paralysis," and "freeze." Read them now more slowly, one at a time, pausing to check your inner body reactions. What happens in your body when you say each of them? What images, body gestures, or responses do you become aware of? How does your posture change, even in subtle ways? You might like to note your results for this mini-practice exercise on the power of words in your pain journal.

In the next chapter, we will build on your connection with your body experience to explore the pain trap that is created by responses to threats of danger that are not released from the body. Since most people in pain are caught in this trap at some point, it's helpful to discover how you may get stuck in it and how to move beyond it.

CHAPTER TWO

The Pain Trap

THE BRAIN RESPONDS to threat by activating certain primitive brain structures, including the brain stem and amygdala, which are involved in maintaining survival. The amygdala, which has been called the smoke detector, or alarm center, of the brain, is central to these reactions. If there is the perception of danger that poses a threat to survival, the amygdala responds by turning on the fear response.

Once the fear response is activated, the body begins to brace to protect itself against threat. For example, our arms may instinctively rise up to protect our heads. Bracing can trigger chronic constriction if it is not released. And if this constriction persists, it creates pain.

Eventually we brace against the pain itself, which creates further constriction and more pain. As this cascade continues, we may also collapse into the helplessness of the freeze response. This vicious cycle or "pain trap" can be self-reinforcing and often difficult to break.

The pain trap deepens in its complexity because the amygdala also shuts down other areas of the brain, such as the frontal lobes, which are essential to our powers of observation, language, and perspective. Because our powers to notice, distance ourselves, and gain perspective from our sensations are diminished when we are in pain that results from fear and other reactions to threat, we begin to believe and experience that we *are* the pain, and we then *become* the pain. Our brains activate this belief, and our experience confirms this because we have no way to process a different reality.

OUT OF THE TRAP TOWARD FREEDOM

To summarize, the pain trap begins when we activate our natural responses in reaction to threats to our survival. These responses are accompanied by the fear response that is turned on by the amygdala, which then activates bracing reactions through the body. First, we brace against the threat that caused the pain and eventually against the internal threat of pain itself. If this cycle of threat → fear → brace → constrict → pain → collapse → threat of pain is not interrupted, many serious problems, including chronic pain, can occur.

To escape this trap, we must shift from "I am the pain" to "I am experiencing the pain" to "I am experiencing the sensations that are underneath the pain." Once we complete these shifts, then we can begin to resolve the pain. We need to regain the ability to observe and to disidentify from the pain, in order to prevent being overpowered and engulfed so completely by our discomfort. To do so, we need to find ways to develop our curiosity and explore the sensations that underlie the pain.

One important intervention is to use the power of curiosity to help interrupt the fear that often marks the first downward slide into the pain trap. As we learn to sustain a playful and mindful focus on the sensations of our bodies, we stop waiting for our worst fears to be fulfilled, and instead begin to discover how our somatic experiences feed into each other and keep the patterns related to threat alive in the present moment.

EXERCISE: Exploring the Felt Sense

The simplest way to explore the felt sense of your body is to start with this moment, whether you're sitting, lying down, or even standing up.

First, get a sense of your feet and how they seem to be (or not be) connected to the earth. For example, are they pressed into the floor, resting on top of a couch or bed, or somehow floating in space? How do you know? Now gently shift your weight from foot to foot. How does this change your awareness?

Next, explore how the rest of your lower body, your calves and thighs, feel connected to your feet. Are there differences between the right and left legs? If so, how would you describe the difference?

Allow your attention to shift to any other part of your body that seems to draw your awareness. What do you notice? What language can help you describe any specific sensations you find? Are you aware instead of a more global sense? How might you describe that?

Once your exploration of a body area seems or feels complete, allow your attention to be drawn to the next part of your body, and so on. For each area, pause to notice your felt sense and then identify the language that might describe how it feels or seems to you.

As you continue, practice using the language of sensation to describe your experience of each area. Examples include: tight, loose, blocked, congested, flowing, tingly, heavy, floating, empty, cold, or warm. Challenge yourself to shift away from thoughts and beliefs. If you notice that you use one sensation word repeatedly, are there other words that can be used more accurately?

If you feel stuck at any time, you can ask yourself: "What kinds of sensations are associated with being stuck? What is this part of my body touching? How does that feel? What smells or tastes am I aware of? Are there any sounds or vibrations I can hear or sense here?"

Is your overall sense of your body right now comfortable, uncomfortable, or neutral? How do you know? How might your felt sense of your body guide you further into types of activity or rest? For example, are you feeling more energized? If so, would you like to take a walk or do some other activity? If you're feeling quiet and calm, can you take more time to explore this resting state? Take a few minutes to record your reactions in your pain notebook.

THE ROLE OF TRAUMA WITH PAIN

Many people are resistant to the idea that their current pain is related to past trauma. We have found that it's very important to communicate this information in ways that each person can accept and work with. Often, we start with a more practical, simplified explanation of the fear-bracing-pain cycle and work with that. Once this basic pattern is resolved, or at least manageable, we often find that images or clues related to past traumatic experiences where the body responded by bracing sometimes begin to surface.

There is a risk of becoming overwhelmed by the perspective that it is necessary to reexamine all the threatening experiences of the past in order to manage pain. We find it's better to work with the basic patterns of pain in present time, and to trust the organism to reveal, through its innate wisdom, the additional somatic sensations and patterns we need to explore for lasting relief.

It is common for people who have significant trauma to become stuck in one or more of the fight, flight, or freeze response patterns, which then determines the types of difficulties that will ensue. For example, many of the soldiers who are coming back from Iraq and other battlefields display symptoms of rage, indicating that they may be stuck in the fight response. Similarly, other returning soldiers exhibit symptoms more related to intense fear, which can stem from incomplete flight responses. With other kinds of trauma, particularly with rape, molestation, and other forms of sexual abuse, particularly if they occur in early childhood, immobilization or freeze may be the main difficulty. Children who have been threatened and molested over time, for example, can present with helplessness, hopelessness, or other depressive symptoms related to the freeze response. Because they could not fight back or escape, they tend to collapse. Often this is associated with feelings of shame and self-blame. This is where a dose of self-compassion can be invaluable.

When first working with chronic pain, it can be useful to focus on the *interaction* of trauma with pain in two main ways. One is to address the trauma that may have begun the pain problem to start with, like an accident or injury, assault, or disease. The other important focus is to realize that pain in and of itself becomes traumatizing.

There is often significant trauma related to the beginning of a pain condition, whether or not there is conscious awareness of this. One of the most dreaded things in the human experience is pain, and the fear that it will become endless and unrelenting. Many older people, for example, have a universal fear, not of dying, but of being in pain. So remember, this is the second arrow in the pain cycle: the recoiling from our sensations that can become a root cause of unnecessary suffering.

Regardless of the nature of the trauma that may be connected to your pain, the principles and practices you will learn in our program will help you unlock its mystery. What we have learned over and over again in working with numerous types of pain is that whenever chronic pain is not resolving even when reasonable treatment has been used, inevitably trauma is the missing link. Once unreleased trauma is identified and liberated from the body, most conditions will then begin to resolve. During the rest of this program, you will learn ways of tracking, working with, and releasing the elements of trauma that may be blocking your progress.

THE INTERFACE OF EMOTIONAL AND PHYSICAL PAIN

As we've suggested earlier in this chapter, it is also important to recognize that working with trauma linked to pain always involves healing both emotional and physical aspects. In fact, it may surprise you to discover that emotional and physical pain operate identically in the brain. With injuries, pain signals often originate from the periphery of the body, but also from parts of the brain related to emotion. Functional brain scans (fMRIs), which measure activity in the brain, have shown that once pain signals reach the brain, three specific areas light up simultaneously: the limbic system (the emotional center), the sensory cortex (which governs sensation), and the cerebral cortex (which organizes thoughts and beliefs).[1]

To summarize, any kind of pain that is ongoing will contain an emotional component, some sensation or physical pain, and various thoughts and beliefs that can block recovery, and which often contribute to pain. In order to resolve any pain condition successfully, it is necessary to work always with the emotional pain aspects, as well as with the physical sensations and the thinking mind's limiting beliefs.

THE IMPORTANCE OF SELF-REGULATION

In our experience, the primary antidote for people who struggle with pain and trauma is to learn how to regulate emotional and sensory experiences, and to calm themselves so the limbic fear and rage systems in the amygdala deactivate. Although the regulatory process is quite complex, we can actually help to restore it with simple awareness practices, such as circle breathing, which we will describe in this next exercise.

EXERCISE: Circle Breathing
◀)) Track 2

Now that you are beginning to understand the wisdom of your felt sense by completing the previous exercise, you can go further to use your breath to open up pathways of movement and flow in your body. These can begin to counteract the constriction of fight, flight, and freeze.

Take a few moments to connect with the overall sense of your body. How would you describe your felt sense of the right side of your body compared to your left? Is there one side of your body that is significantly less comfortable than the other? Pause briefly and use the language of sensation to describe the felt sense of each side of your body. You may find sensations such as heavy, light, tight, burning, loose, and aching, among others.

Now imagine that you can breathe in through the more comfortable side of your body, starting with your foot and lower leg on that side, and progressing up to the area where it feels like your breathing connects with the core of your body (usually through your belly in the center of your body). Then sense your breath as it crosses your belly or diaphragm to the other side of your body. As you exhale, imagine that your breath moves down and through the other leg and foot and out into the earth. Repeat this three to four times, noticing your felt sense of what is different in your body each time.

Next, imagine that your breath is a magnet that can pick up the more comfortable sensations (name them as you breathe) so that as you breathe in, up the more comfortable side of your body, your breath picks up these sensations and shifts them over through your belly, and then down and through the less comfortable side of your body, and through your leg and foot into the earth. Again, pause and notice what is different now in the felt sense of your body experience. For example, do you feel lighter, more energized, more calm, less tense or tight, or do you experience some other kind of change? What is it?

If this exercise does not seem to be helping you shift in the direction of flow and ease, imagine breathing up the more uncomfortable side of the body this time, letting your breath cross over through your belly. Then imagine breathing down and out through the more comfortable side of the body. What difference does this make? What is your felt sense now of your lower body? Of your upper body? Of your body as a whole?

If both sides of your body feel equally comfortable or uncomfortable, or you want to try another variation of circle breathing, practice breathing up the middle (midline) of your body, imagining that your inhale starts at the base of your pelvis and rises up to your nose and face. Then imagine you can breathe out, down, and through both sides of your body, through both your shoulders, arms, and hands, and down through both your legs and out through your feet. Repeat this process for three to four breath cycles. What is this like for you?

Finally, if your problem area is in your cervical, thoracic, or lumbar spine, or you want more practice with this technique, imagine that you can breathe up the middle front of your body to the top of your head. As you breathe out, sense your breath moving down the back of your head, neck, mid-back, and through your lower back and out through your tailbone; finally, imagine it cascading down both of your legs. Repeat this several times. What are the effects? How are they different from the first three steps of practicing circle breathing? [2]

Remember to record your observations from this exercise in your pain journal.

Equally important to regulating the emotional and sensory elements of body experience is to focus on strengthening social engagement and building a support system to help with self-regulation. This should include a secure relationship with treatment professionals. Throughout the rest of this program, we will explore many of the specific self-regulation tools we have found most useful, along with tips for building collaborative and supportive relationships with yourself and others.

In addition to learning to use social support, you will also learn specific tools to deactivate and counteract some of the common factors that often bridge from normal acute pain into the downward spiral of chronic pain. This process, explained in our next chapter, will help you begin to free yourself from the pain trap and lead you forward on the path of ultimate freedom from pain.

CHAPTER THREE

Neutralizing the Factors That Cause Chronic Pain

IN CHAPTER 2, we explored the concept that if our natural reactions to threats are not completed and released from the body, the accumulation of ongoing bracing and defensive reactions related to fight, flight, and freeze can generate continued pain, resulting in a pain trap.

This chapter will discuss how the shift occurs from normal, necessary pain to more chronic pain that persists after the initial cause of the pain has resolved. Self-regulation can fail for all of the "big three" trauma reactions—fight, flight, and freeze—through the mechanisms of:

- dissociation
- anxiety, fear, and panic
- helplessness and hopelessness
- anger, rage, and irritability

We will discuss each of these, and offer you a toolbox for working with them and breaking free of pain entrapment.

DISSOCIATION

The first type of shift we'll explore occurs through the defense of dissociation, which is connected to the freeze response. Dissociation is the most primitive element of our natural response to pain, as well as to threat and trauma. It's a kind of automatic disconnection from the environment as a whole. It allows us to deal with overwhelming anxiety and fear by minimizing movement and the expenditure of energy as well as by numbing so that we do not feel pain.

If you've ever been in even a minor vehicular accident, you know firsthand how this works. You can be driving along in the flow of traffic, listening to music, registering the scenery flashing by, aware of your own thoughts, daydreams, and memories. In the next moment you can be plunged into the darkness of fear and uncertainty, as well as the disorienting aftereffects of a punishing impact with another vehicle. You may be able to check your body for obvious injury, get out of the car, check with the other driver, and retrieve and exchange information. You may possibly even be able to tell your story to a police officer or paramedic called to the scene (as Bill was able to do, even with a head trauma).

At some point in this process, however, you may notice that you do not actually feel your body, so, in fact, you cannot be a fully reliable witness of your own injuries. This numbing is due to the shock response and the protective activation of chemicals, such as endorphins, turned on by various centers of the brain. These chemicals are designed to minimize pain so that appropriate defensive action can take place. Dissociation is actually a vital survival skill. When dissociation becomes habitual, however, the dissociated person gets lost in this condition and cannot find the way back to a more connected state.

The Way Back

If you are significantly dissociated from your body, including its pain responses, the first step to coming out of shock (whether recent or longstanding) is to begin to sense when and how you're dissociated, and then learn to gradually reconnect with your body. As you reconnect, you will discover and build various types of resources that will help you to resolve your body's stress and pain responses. We call this self-regulation. The ability to achieve successful self-regulation of your body's stress responses will lead to less reliance on dissociation, faster resolution of pain, and a greater sense of empowerment and strength.

Shifting Dissociation

There are many tools that can help you begin to decrease your dissociation, so that you can reconnect with and begin to explore your body experience (including your pain) in a safe, productive way. In this part of the chapter, we will introduce you to several necessary skills and tools, while also giving you opportunities to practice them.

One starting place is to find out what you experience in the dissociated state. Sometimes this can be the kind of classic dissociation, where you perceive that, "I'm outside my body; I'm looking down at the room; I see you; I see me." If you are aware of detaching, it's important to notice *how* you're detaching, by expanding the experience of it. For example, if the detachment begins to feel like a floating sensation, an expansion of this experience might lead to the question: "Do I feel like I'm floating more to the right or more to the left, or in some other direction?" Then, can you describe what you see from that place?

Next, after expanding the experience from outside your body, try to describe what you are aware of *in* your body—even if this is very tenuous. Within a few moments, you may have the astonishing experience of coming back into your body and returning to yourself, with your anxiety and fear significantly reduced. The key is always to follow your felt sense, as best as you can, through the dissociation. This is something that has to be a slow, gentle, stepwise process so that you experience a "return home" to the knowledge that it's OK to come back into your body.

As you read this, you might react to this suggestion with a comment like, "But I don't feel anything. I'm just numb." Whether you're aware of it or not, there has to be a part of your body that feels less numb than any other part. In this situation, you can use a body scan,[1] focusing methodically from the top of the head to the bottom of the feet to track your body experience more carefully. This way you will find differences, even if they are small or subtle ones.

To perform and experience a *body scan,* take a few minutes right now to focus on your body experience. Begin either at the top of your head or with the bottom of your feet. Gently "sense in" to the area you have chosen, becoming aware of various types of sensations. If you "don't feel anything," ask yourself what it's like to feel nothing, and note your response.

Then move on to the next area that you sense. From the top of your head, you might move down into your face, jaw, and the sides of your head. If you started at the bottom of your feet, consider what it's like to find and focus on the tops of your feet and on your lower legs. What sensations do you find here?

Continue to flow through various areas of your body somewhat systematically, finding a rhythm with how and where you move from place to place. When the experience feels complete, what feels different in your relationship with your body as compared with when you started this practice? (For more extensive information and practice about body scans, please refer to page 166 in the resource section).

Toolbox for Shifting Dissociation

If you are experienced in working with your body, you may wonder if the tools in this section are too basic for you. We ask that you experiment with them, even though you might think you know what will happen. Both of us regularly use these tools ourselves, and consistently make important discoveries that add to our body resources, sometimes in unexpected and creative ways.

Mindfulness

A primary self-help skill that will support your reconnection to your body is to develop mindfulness in order to become a better observer of your body experience. One important way of engaging mindfulness is to develop awareness of a relatively neutral or comfortable place in your body that is reliable across time. In other words, whenever you become upset, over-activated, or disconnected, it's very helpful to find the place in your body that brings you a consistent sense of connection and a relative sense of security and safety. Finding even a neutral somatic experience that evokes feelings of security, no matter what is going on inside you or around you, is often very effective.

The following exercise will encourage you to develop the resource of rest in your body by finding a place (or a series of places) that can serve as a refuge for you from pain and discomfort.

EXERCISE: Securing a Resting Place in Your Body
🔊)) Track 3

Starting at your head or feet (whichever you prefer), gradually journey to areas where you find some degree of "OK-ness" in your body—not necessarily positive sensations, but not painful ones either. Then, pay attention to the parts of your body that you cannot feel—those that are numb or blank. These may be areas from which you consistently disconnect, such as your feet and legs, hands and fingers, chest or pelvis. Notice whether they seem connected with past injury or areas of habitual stress.

Take a few moments to use your breath and sense your way into one of the numb or disconnected locations you have chosen. Breathing in, feel that part of your body; while breathing out, feel that part of your body again. After three to four breath cycles, ask yourself, "What am I sensing in that area now? Does this part of my body feel more connected? Less connected? Is my sense of it shifting in a positive direction?"

Come back to this exercise again either later on in the same day or another day. Has your sense of this part of your body changed? In what ways does it feel neutral? Does it offer more comfort over time? How does your connection with this place in your body change your pain?

Note your experience with this and the other exercises in your pain journal to maximize your results.

Grounding

Another simple resource to help you shift out of dissociation is grounding through your feet and legs. This next exercise will help you learn to feel grounded as a way of staying centered in relation to pain.

Grounding is one of the foundational skills in learning to connect with your body. Grounding generally involves balancing the energy in your body by connecting with the gravitational forces that hold us securely on the earth. Grounding exercises, such as the one we've recorded on track 4, will help you link with physical and spiritual, mental and emotional energies, bringing them into alignment, and making it safe for you to inhabit your body.

In a way, grounding is similar to electrical grounding, which connects electrical circuits to the earth, allowing energy to move safely into the earth and preventing mechanical damage, fire, or other negative effects. Lightning rods, for example, are grounding devices that allow the electricity of lightning to pass safely from the air into the earth without damaging humans or property.

Grounding processes, like the one we are guiding you through in this exercise, allow you to connect fully with your body without stressing or overwhelming your energy circuits. They will also help you engage with your legs and feet so as to provide a solid foundation for exploring the rest of your body.

EXERCISE: Grounding
🔊)) Track 4

First, begin by gently shifting your weight from foot to foot. Perhaps imagine that they are like the suction cups on a frog's foot connecting you firmly, but flexibly, to the ground.

Next, while breathing in, press gently, through one or both legs, into the floor. While breathing out, let go of the tension in your body. Experiment with how much tension you can release while still being able to hold yourself up in a stable way. Now try the reverse. Breathe in and feel the flow of breath coming into your body, then while breathing out, press gently into the floor through one or both legs.

How do the sensations of pressing down, alternating with letting go, help you feel more connected with your body? Experiment with decreasing or increasing the pressure through your feet and legs until you feel a positive sense of connection. How does grounding affect your sense of well-being?

Don't forget to note your experience with this exercise in your pain journal. ✍

Breathing

Another resource to shift out of disconnection and dissociation is to keep a sustained focus on breathing. Rather than trying to control or change how you breathe, our goal is to teach you awareness of the actual experience of breathing. Often, just taking this simple step results in a shift of tension and pain. If nothing else, your awareness of breathing will usually result in a feeling of greater connectedness to yourself and to others.

EXERCISE: Just One Breath
🔊)) Track 5

Without consciously trying to change your breathing, simply follow the sense of your breath as it moves in and through your body, and again as your breath moves out, just like waves lapping on the beach flow in and out. What changes in your body during that one inhale/exhale cycle? What changes in your pain?

If this is helpful, follow the pathway of a second breath as it moves through your body, as it comes in, and then as it goes out, again sensing it like the tides of the ocean that ebb and flow. What changes in your body this time? What further changes in your pain do you notice?

Feel free to come back to this exercise again and again.[2] Use it whenever you are aware of anxiety, stress, or discomfort.

One important distinction we emphasize is that the focus of the breathing practice is not as much on inhaling, but on exhaling. In other words, it is essential to learn to allow a full exhalation rather than to focus on creating a full inhalation. The next exercise will help you practice extending your out-breath.

Tibetan and other spiritually guided chants have been used successfully for thousands of years to facilitate healing and open the doors of perception. We borrowed this exercise, with certain modifications, from these chants. The "voo" sound will open, expand, and vibrate the organs in the belly. This vibration, in turn, may stimulate the vagus nerve (the largest nerve in the body after the spinal cord) and will provide new signals that can help a shutdown or overstimulated nervous system to rebalance. This simple exercise can make a real difference in your relationship to pain, sometimes shifting your pain dramatically, and other times creating a more gradual shift.

EXERCISE: Voo Breathing
🔊)) Track 6

Begin the exercise by finding a comfortable place to sit. Slowly inhale a full breath, then pause momentarily. On your out-breath, gently vibrate the sound "voo," as though the sound were coming from your belly. Sustain this sound throughout the whole exhalation. Let the breath go all the way out, and then pause, waiting for the next breath to come in on its own. If you like, repeat this several times. Then feel your body, particularly your fingers, hands, and feet, as well as any other parts of your body that feel enlivened or reduced in pain.

You can do this exercise as many times a day as you want. We suggest doing it at least three times a day, especially when you begin to feel stress or when your pain starts to increase. You can also use this at the end of the day when you're lying in bed and about to go to sleep—and then in the morning (along with a cat-like stretch) to greet the new day.

Record your experience with this exercise in your pain journal, noting how you feel after you use it in a variety of circumstances.

Positive Regulation of Your Breathing

For some people, over-focusing on breathing can be a problem if they attempt to control their breathing. Controlled breathing is generally only helpful for a breath or two; for example, if you're in a state of panic or intense anxiety and you want to calm yourself just for the moment, you might take a few deep, easy breaths—accenting the out-breath. Try this next exercise to help you find a different kind of spontaneous regulation of your breathing.

EXERCISE: Modified Diaphragmatic Breathing

Place one hand on top of the other just above your belly button. While inhaling, press down gently with both hands, and then while exhaling, let all the muscles in your belly relax or loosen, including those in the hands.

You may want to experiment with reversing this breathing practice. To do this, keep one hand over the other on your diaphragm and press down gently while you exhale, letting all muscles relax when you breathe in. Continue for several breath cycles. What differences do you find in the results between the two approaches?

Some people also find it helpful to add grounding through the feet or legs to this practice. If you'd like to try this, press gently through your feet and legs at the same time you are pressing down gently with your hands on your diaphragm (either during the inhale or exhale, whichever you prefer). Notice how this feels.

What do you discover as you do this exercise? Within a few seconds, many people discover that those feelings of connection with their breathing and their bodies increase. As always, if the exercise does not feel helpful, please discontinue it for the time being.

Please note your experience with this exercise in your pain journal. ✐

An important caveat is that, for some people, just focusing on their breathing can lead to more anxiety, especially if the breathing practice is unguided. If this occurs for you, circle breathing (see exercise on page 24) can be a better alternative. This is because the focus is more on the periphery of the body and not on the diaphragm, belly, or core. Remember, it is always a matter of what works best for you. It's essential to feel full permission to experiment, and if a technique or practice isn't working, let it go and move on. There are many other techniques that may be more appropriate, more timely, and more effective for you.

ANXIETY, FEAR, AND PANIC

Another of the most common sets of reactions to trauma and pain consists of anxiety. Generalized anxiety is diagnosed when there is chronic, exaggerated worry and tension. And even though there's seemingly nothing that provokes it (or alternatively, everything provokes it), there can be very clear symptoms.

One set of symptoms is related to the sympathetic branch of the central nervous system and includes restlessness, feeling keyed up, or on edge. Other symptoms include feeling easily fatigued, especially as the situation becomes more and more chronic. Also, there can be difficulty with concentration, disturbance of thoughts or awareness, or problems associated with blanking out mentally. General irritability, muscle tension, and sleep disturbance constitute yet another set of difficulties. The latter category can include difficulty falling asleep or staying asleep. Panic, in contrast, is usually associated with strong somatic sensations such as a racing, pounding heart, difficulty breathing, shortness of breath, or a queasy twisted gut.

What we can conclude from neurobiological research is that panic and fear are triggered by the amygdala, our "all-points bulletin" natural alarm center. Trauma disrupts our alarm system through the mechanism of memory. Past traumatic events are stored in procedural or implicit memory as though they were ongoing and still happening at the present time.[3]

The result is an alarm system that seems to be randomly firing, but is actually firing due to unconscious cues from the past. We end up with a perpetual warning that something is wrong, that we're always in danger. So we can have nearly constant activation from fragmentary emotional memories that impair our thinking brains. That is why we can't intervene very well when we are having an anxiety or panic response.

In addition, pain can intensify greatly when the nervous system, over-activated by fear, goes rogue. Nerves begin to send out false alarms due to the development of *pain hypersensitivity*. This hypersensitivity can cause even benign sensory experiences, such as the touch of cloth on skin, to be triggering and painful. When this happens, pain ceases to be adaptive and becomes an illness in and of itself, creating persistent, unceasing torment.

Some individuals with unresolved trauma seem to experience more of a terror or fear response first thing in the morning, while others report this surge in the evening. Although we don't know exactly what causes this phenomenon, we suspect that it's due to fluctuating cortisol levels. It's been widely accepted that people suffering from chronic PTSD have low cortisol levels, due to its depletion over time from heightened amygdala response.[4]

A research study of individuals involved in self-harm cutting[5] indicated that cortisol levels were very, very low on the first day, then increased gradually, until on the seventh day the subjects exhibited

relatively high cortisol levels. At the high point of the cycle, partici-
pants tended to cut themselves. What seemed to help them was to ask
that they not get out of bed immediately to avoid their anxiety, but
begin to make small stretching movements instead.

Toolbox for Shifting Anxiety, Fear, and Panic

Moving Just a Little Bit

When most people wake up in an anxious state, they tend either to stay in
that state or they try to jump up and occupy themselves with something
else. If you tend to wake up with high anxiety, try moving just a little bit.
You might practice some of the breathing exercises that have already worked
for you in this program. Then, slowly get out of bed and begin to mobilize more gradually by doing your regular morning activities at a relatively
slow pace. Periodically, you may want to sit for a little while and evaluate
how the anxiety feels and how you feel in general. This kind of self-paced
approach seems to result in more stabilized cortisol levels and less fear.

Islands of Safety

Many people in pain are aware that as soon as their pain levels increase, they
fall into states of anguish and anxiety. This reflects the intimate relationship that exists between pain and anxiety. In this program, we present a
number of tools that work effectively with anxiety related to pain, and with
pain related to anxiety. The key is to find what works best at a given time.
Sometimes even an hour or perhaps a day later, the solution may change.

One effective strategy is to build "islands of safety." When you find
yourself in a raging sea of trauma, anxiety, fear, or pain, you may find a
tiny island where you can settle, if only for a moment's rest. One idea
is to find the resting place in your body that you discovered in the first
exercise in this chapter, Securing a Resting Place in Your Body (page
31). Repeat the exercise now and find a resting place or refuge from
pain or discomfort. From there you can search for another tiny island.

Then perhaps, you can create a bridge between these islands. As you continue along, you can begin to assemble a real landmass, a large solid island, which may have hills and an interior.

The key to working with these very difficult states of fear, of anguish, of helplessness, is to learn tools that can change your experience even a little bit. The nervous system really can't change too much at once, particularly in chronic situations. But if you can achieve one small shift here, and then another there, eventually you discover that you're on stable ground, and that the raging sea of pain and stress is going on around you, but you're not in the middle of it anymore; you're settled on the safety of an island instead.

Pause, Take One Breath, and Choose

Another idea is to find relief from anxiety through a simple three-step model. When you become aware of an increase in pain or anxiety, the first and most important step is to pause. Really get a sense of pausing and slowing everything down.

The next step is to take one breath with full awareness (see the Just One Breath exercise on page 33). Notice what happens in your body as you take only one full breath.

After that one breath—and you may want or need to take several more—you will then be in a position where you can make choices. You can choose to explore the possibility of islands of safety, of gentle stretching and movement, or use other tools based on breathing, mindfulness, or energy psychology, or any of the other techniques presented in this program. Just taking that one breath may set you in motion beyond fear, pain, and trauma.

Resolving More Lasting States of Anxiety, Fear, and Panic

Focus on resolving anxiety and fear states needs to take place throughout treatment of pain. We believe that all chronic pain conditions are also anxiety conditions—that is, pain is intimately related to the experience of dysregulated fear, when fear causes the body to constrict or brace against the pain. This causes the organism to experience more pain, which then triggers more fear and anxiety, and so forth.

One important way to work with fear is through mindful observation. When we are able to stand at a distance from fear, observe it, and take it apart as physical sensation along with its related thoughts and images, the fear often dissolves and transforms.

To get a sense of how this works, imagine that you are able to flee the source of your pain. If there's an incident that started your pain, like an accident or injury, imagine that you can run away from that scene.

Joe, for example, imagined that he could sense the impact that caused the motorcycle accident that left him with chronic back pain before it actually happened. He envisioned revving up his engine and directing his bike safely in a different direction, then feeling the sense of successful escape in his body.

If there is a scene for you that is connected to the onset of your pain, imagine that you can use your legs to run away, or jump and roll out of harm's way, or otherwise execute a planned escape. What do you feel in your body as you imagine this? How do you experience the flight response? What effect does this have on your memory of the incident? What effect does it have on your pain now? You might want to note your reactions to this mini-exercise in your pain journal.

HELPLESSNESS AND HOPELESSNESS

Helplessness comes from being overwhelmed by anxiety and fear. If you're not overwhelmed, you may be able to experience fear, or even terror, without a long-lasting effect, because you know somehow that you're going to be able to move through it. But when people don't have this experience of knowing that they will be able to move through anxiety, chaos, and fear, this can lead to sensations, feelings, and postures of helplessness and of hopelessness.

Much of the research on helplessness has been done by psychologist Dr. Marty Seligman, who developed the term "learned helplessness"[6] to refer to a situation where we perceive that we have no choices, or no control, over the outcome of very difficult, in some cases, life-threatening circumstances. Robert Scaer has suggested in his book *The Trauma Spectrum* that helplessness and hopelessness may be related to an unresolved freeze response.[7]

Toolbox for Shifting Helplessness and Hopelessness

We invite you to experience a series of tools to help you resolve helplessness and collapse. Take your time to explore these possibilities, working with one or more that seem to resonate for you. If none of them appeal to you, or if they feel overwhelming in any way, feel free to leave them for now and return at another time.

Working with the Posture of Helplessness

Helplessness and resignation are embodied as a collapsed posture—the shoulders slumped forward, the chest caved in, a folding around the area of the diaphragm (midriff). The posture is one of giving up. So in helping people begin to become aware of those postures, we often work with them in a standing position. When you're standing up, your muscles have to deal with gravity, and can't completely collapse. If they are sitting down, collapse can occur far more easily. Here's an exercise you can use to find out how to explore the sensations and feelings of helplessness.

EXERCISE: Shifting the Posture of Helplessness and Collapse
◀)) Track 7

While standing up, notice the parts of your body that feel strong in some way. Maybe you notice strength in your ankles, legs, thighs, arms, elbows, or shoulders. Pay attention to sensations in those areas that are even a little bit different from helplessness and collapse. Spend a little time exploring the sense of strength throughout your body, mapping and affirming those areas of improvement using the language of sensation. In your pain journal, note your experience of discovering your strengths.

Another important step is to notice in daily life whenever you start to experience the feeling or sense of helplessness. This might be related to your pain or some other challenge. If possible, go to a mirror and notice your posture. See if you can recognize specific places where your posture seems or feels collapsed, and then continue by practicing a few simple movements to begin to shift it. Remember to record your experience with the posture of helplessness in your pain journal. ✎

Connecting with Conflict-Free Experience

Another way of working with this type of collapse into helplessness can be accomplished by connecting with conflict-free experience[8] in your body. This technique refers to finding areas where you don't experience helplessness, pain, or self-blame reactions.

EXERCISE: Connecting with Conflict-Free Experience
🔊 Track 8

A simple way to find conflict-free experience is to ask yourself, "When, in the last day or so, have I felt least anxious or least in pain, and most like the self I hope to embody most of the time?" You may not be completely free of pain in this kind of moment, but there are always moments when you feel a little less pain, for example when you are laughing with a friend, taking a walk, or during other times of simple, pleasant engagement.

When you find that moment, see if you can represent that experience in your mind's eye—as an image or a thought. Then shift back and forth between that image (or thought) and your body sensations. As you do this, notice how your body may be containing or holding the experience that is free of conflict, anxiety, pain, or helplessness. Then use your attention to go back and forth between your image or memory of the experience, and whatever sense of it you have in your body.

Repeat these steps two or three times, and then think of another time a week or two ago that was relatively conflict free. What do you notice? How can you describe the sensations in your body that result from this practice? Now think of another moment when you felt less pain and more freedom. Explore the felt sense of this moment. What happens to your pain as you practice? Note your experience with this tool in your pain journal. ✐

Techniques to Reduce Negative Feelings before Searching Out Conflict-Free Moments

Another strategy is to use various techniques to lower anxiety, panic, or helplessness *before* finding a conflict-free moment. One example of how to do this is to use a technique (derived from applied kinesiology) often used in the practice of Energy Psychology called the "over-energy correction" or Cook's Hookup.[9] From this point of view, panic, fear, and anxiety all involve a situation in which too much energy is trying to flow through your energy pathways or meridians. There's a lack of containment and a lack of flow.

If you've never encountered this type of approach before, be forewarned that it can seem a little strange and unfamiliar. Yet many people have good results with it in terms of reducing anxiety or fear—so if you're ready for an "out of your usual box" experience, give it a try.

EXERCISE: Over-Energy Correction

To practice this technique, while sitting or lying down, cross your left ankle over your right if you are right-handed (reverse the directions if you're left-handed). Then stretch your arms in front of you so that they're parallel to the floor (if you are lying down, just reach toward the ceiling), with the backs of your two hands touching each other. Next, cross your right hand over your left and clasp your fingers together, fold your hands and arms, drawing your fingers down and back toward you, eventually pointing your fingers toward your face.

Rest your hands and elbows on your chest. If you are at all uncomfortable in your wrists or your arms, modify this position by just crossing your arms over your chest with your right arm over your left (See more specifics including a diagram under "Energy Approaches," page 168, in the resources section).

Then place your tongue at the back of your upper front teeth, on the palate. Close your mouth and eyes, and just breathe for a few moments. Usually within the first ten seconds there begins to be a shift. Notice what happens for you, and continue for as long as your response is positive.

Many people report a deep settling into their bodies with a sense of calm. If this works for you, you can use this approach before you go to bed at night or if you wake up and are not able to return easily to sleep. You can also use it to manage many kinds of anxiety-fear responses including panic.

Note your experience with this exercise in your pain journal. ✑

As with any technique, pay attention to your experience so that you can make nurturing choices in selecting those tools that have positive or neutral effects. As we have said before, this program includes many alternative possibilities so that you can find and choose the methods that are most effective for you.

ANGER, RAGE, AND IRRITABILITY

Every day we have stresses that frustrate us and trigger anger. A driver pulls sharply in front of us without warning and we slam on the brakes, narrowly avoiding a collision, and the papers we had on the front seat are thrown all over the floor. Later in the day, a coworker repeats a mistake for the fifth time in a row, even after promising to resolve the issue. That evening, we learn that our spouse or partner has forgotten, once again, to complete a promised financial transaction, missing a deadline and incurring late fees.

Whether we want to or not, we have predictable reactions to these kinds of situations: elevated heartbeat, flushing, or the feeling that an internal volcano is about to erupt.

Anger is a normal reaction and can stimulate us to take action in adverse situations. It is related to the third of the "big three" reactions to pain and threat—the unreleased fight response. Like flight and freeze, fight reactions are important survival options when we are threatened with danger. When the fight mode is turned on through our body's alarm system, powerful chemicals are released to give us more energy to persist in the face of obstacles, to ward off attacks, and even to counterattack.

Feeling anger can serve an enlivening function, empowering us to stay strong instead of collapsing into helplessness. It's also a normal reaction when we lose basic trust in other people, because this is yet another type of threat to our sense of safety and security. Like the other survival responses, however, problems occur when the fight response is continually activated in the present moment due to reminders of past threats. When the energy of the fight response is not completed or released in appropriate action or discharge, it can create intense muscle tension, inflammation, and other systemic reactions that contribute significantly to pain. When feelings of anger or rage go unmanaged, they can trigger fierce reactions that are out of proportion to current realities, creating fear at the power of our angry reactions, whether provoked or not.

The problem here is not anger. The problem is that we often don't know how to cope with, or express, feelings of anger in a fruitful way. We are also confused by other companion feelings such as resentment, hurt, frustration, disappointment, jealousy, and shame. Anger is simply a natural instinctive response to obstacles in our path and to many different circumstances where we feel powerless or victimized.

However, the habitual ways we express angry feelings and the energy of the fight response may be counterproductive. If we are unable to express our anger effectively, our automatic "short fuse" reactions may trigger us to react with full activation as if our circumstances were actually life threatening, causing problems in our work and family relationships. Continually angry individuals may actually provoke others to react aggressively and with hostility toward them, because of the inflexible ways they attempt to control their environments. This can set up a self-fulfilling prophecy associated with trauma-related beliefs like "I can't trust anyone," or "After all I've been through, I deserve to be treated better than this," or "Why didn't so-and-so prepare me for what could happen?"

Any effective treatment of pain should include awareness that fight responses are always present, as are freeze and flight reactions, whether or not they are being expressed. And as with any persistent discomfort, pain itself can activate arousal of the fight response since we can become angry at the events that created the pain to begin with, angry that our pain is unmanageable, angry that no one can protect us from the suffering that pain provokes. Additionally, if we have been significantly threatened or abused at a young age, we may not have learned flexible, effective ways to respond to conflict.

Somatic Contours of Emotional Anger

As emphasized in chapter 1, all pain conditions have sensate, emotional, and cognitive components. Discussion of anger, and the fight response, gives us the ideal opportunity to examine the wedding between emotion and sensation. Similar interfaces exist between fear reactions and the flight response, and between helplessness and collapse related to the freeze response.

We have said that the pain trap is created by the vicious cycle of bracing against the threat of danger, possible injury, or further pain; which leads, in turn, to constriction and more pain and fear, and so on. We can also become trapped by anger responses that become too compulsive, rigid, easily triggered, or explosive.

The primary intervention to prevent imprisonment in any of these traps is through the use of body awareness to process the emotional component of a threat response *just as it is* in the body. If we experience anger in its purest form in any given moment, free from mental analysis and judgment, we can begin to "dismantle" our habitual responses and enter into new, and energizing, somatic experience. In other words, when we access our feelings through carefully paced body awareness, rather than through rapid cathartic emotional release, we are able to create the lasting change in emotional patterns that we desire.

Toolbox for Regulating Anger, Rage, and Irritability

There are numerous tools that can help you effectively regulate your anger and fight responses. Try one or more of the following options and, as always, enter into an attitude of curious exploration so that you can move on if you aren't satisfied with the results.

Shifting Habitual Anger Patterns

Learning how we deal with and resolve prolonged states of anger and rage has enormous impact on our abilities to transition to a pain-free life. Since these emotions trigger terror of our own aggression, we often turn these feelings in on ourselves because we are too afraid of expressing—or even feeling—them. The exercises that follow will teach you how to track, contain, and safely express these powerful emotions and their related sensations.

EXERCISE: Free Yourself from Habitual Anger and Rage

> *Tracking Bodily Sensations.* The first step in shifting destructive emotional patterns is to track the bodily sensations that underlie the anger. Take a moment to think of a situation that frequently triggers anger, irritability, or frustration for you. Notice what happens

in your body. You may become distracted by negative thoughts related to the anger response, but don't be distracted by their content or your analysis. Instead return to and stay with the sensations in your body.

At first this may be confusing or distressing because it's so different from your usual focus. However, as you hold these sensations in your awareness, without trying to change anything, feeling them just as they are, eventually your body experience will seem more spacious and settled. This is because as the underlying sensations of anger become uncoupled or separated from the emotion and then unhooked from related thoughts or beliefs, and even from images or memory, the felt sense becomes more fluid, moving toward subtler, freer "contours" of feeling.

What happens right now as you stay with the sensations of your anger? Note your experience in your pain journal. What part of your body wants to express anger when you think of the anger trigger you selected a moment ago? What part seems afraid of the anger and wants to hold it back? Remember, the feeling of anger evolves from the fight response of wanting to strike out and attack. This holding back accumulates in our bodies as muscle tension and pain, and prevents the expression of healthy aggression.

Containing Powerful Feelings. To befriend your anger, you will also need to learn how to contain, or hold within you, powerful feelings. When we give into our usual ways of dealing with anger (which is either to stuff or suppress it or mindlessly express it), we are often trying to release the tension and feel relief from the powerful emotional charge. However, this may make no lasting change in our capacity to tap into the positive, life-affirming energy of anger.

To feel what healthy aggression is like, take a really crisp apple and take a big bite out of it. Now chew it with great vigor. Then take another big bite, enjoying the crunch and the power of your teeth biting down and destroying the apple by pulverizing it. Finally, take in the juicy nourishment of the fruit. This is what pure healthy aggression feels like.

Examine Your Reactions in the Past. Think of a time in the past when you actually expressed your full anger at another person. Maybe you shook your fist, raised your voice, exploded into swear words, shoved him or her, or pointed your finger.

What was the effect of your behavior on the other person and on yourself? Notice as you explore the answer to this question whether you become more connected with anger or less connected.

What did you learn? What do you think might happen the next time you encounter a similar situation? ✐

Explore The Roots of the Fight Response

To continue your study of the fight response, it can be useful to feel the animal roots of this powerful response to threat.

EXERCISE: Exploring the Roots of the Fight Response
◀)) Track 9

Imagine that you are your favorite wild animal—strong, powerful, and quick—whatever appeals to you at the moment you are reading this.

Feel the sense of your strength and power in your animal body. What sensations do you notice? Now stand up and begin to walk around the room. Let your eyes narrow so that you can get a sense of deliberate movement as you, more and more, "step into" the body of this animal. How do you experience your strength, power, and forcefulness?

Now imagine that another animal is approaching. You know, instinctively, that this animal is also strong and powerful; it is a force to reckon with, just as you are. You also sense that this animal wants to attack you. What do you begin to feel in your body? If you sense that you are going to collapse or shrink back, remember that this is your territory and that you have a right to defend it. What are the sensations that signal your determination to protect what is yours? Pay particular attention to sensations of determination and strength in your head, neck, shoulders, face, and jaw. What movements and tensions do you feel? What emotions are you aware of? Feel the strength in your shoulders, arms, legs, and feet.

Finally, prepare to take action toward the animal that is trying to invade your space and usurp what is yours. Notice what happens as you prepare to fight back and to protect your vital interests. Follow those sensations and movements, staying grounded in your body's felt sense of your own animal power and strength. Feel how your shoulders, arms, and neck tense as you prepare to strike out. Does the energy related to fight begin to shift? If so, how? Continue to stay with these sensations until you sense completion. What does completion feel like? What happens to your pain?

Become Aware of the Feelings of Healthy Aggression

The following exercise can help you process anger about an event in the past as well as work with current anger reactions.

EXERCISE: Working with Healthy Aggression
◀)) Track 10

First, constrict your hand into a fist and clench it tight. This act can represent being locked up in anger. You might even want to name the

50

resentments, irritations, and anger that you're aware of, and sense your fist clenching tighter and tighter to hold onto the anger.

Now gradually open your hand and extend your fingers so that they're mostly straight but also form a bit of a cup. Where did the anger go? The lesson is that if you can learn to let go of anger in your body, it will tend to dissolve, or even "disappear," because its energy is transformed in the letting go.

Now make your hand into a fist again, and again gradually allow it to open. What sensations are you aware of as your hand continues to open? Name all the ones you are experiencing. What do you notice as you practice using the language of sensation to describe your experience?

Explore the Sensations Underneath Anger

Often when we surrender to the urge to get angry, we simply let off steam like a pressure cooker. This does not allow us, however, to find ways of turning down the heat so that we can regulate the underlying buildup of anger (or steam). This next exercise teaches you how to feel the underlying sensations.

EXERCISE: Feeling the Sensations Underneath Anger

Start with a feeling of anger toward someone in your life. Feel and name the sensations as you track each one from its starting point to a sense of completion, change, or stuckness. Resist the temptation to detour by getting into your thought process.

If you feel stuck, just track your breathing as you focus on the anger. Feel the rhythm of the rise and release of your chest, the wave of energy and where and how it moves through your upper body. Stay with the sense of movement, the feel of muscles expanding and then letting go.

As you sense your somatic experience beginning to shift, return your attention to the anger you began to explore. What is different now? If you envision the next time you're likely to experience the same kind of irritability, frustration, or anger, can you imagine shifting your attention to your sensations and breathing whenever you feel blocked or stuck, and then returning and expressing your anger with words meant to connect rather than to distance?

Jot down your experiences in your pain journal, then return to this exercise at a later time when you are feeling triggered by anger. What happens over time as you practice this approach?

The next chapter will help you continue on the journey from uncontrollable or unmanageable emotional or physical pain, which can result from insufficient self-regulation, back to the place of stable functioning. As in the current chapter, you will encounter additional practice exercises to help you develop specific skills in self-regulation that lead to further wholeness, balance, and stability. Our message will continue to show you how your unresolved stress reactions to threat and trauma can serve as the pathway to transforming your pain condition through the use of simple tools we present.

CHAPTER FOUR

The Journey Back from Unmanageable Pain

IN THIS CHAPTER, we will examine the basic journey back to full recovery and how you can work with the obstacles that challenge that movement. Although each person's return from unregulated pain to hard-won stability is unique, we have found that this journey consists of three general stages:

1. self-regulation
2. transformation
3. resilience, continued recovery, and restoration of the deep self

We will discuss the first two stages in this chapter, while stage three will be discussed in chapter 6.

STAGE ONE: ACHIEVING RELIABLE SELF-REGULATION

In order to complete the first stage of achieving reliable self-regulation, you will learn to strengthen the skills begun in the first two chapters and add additional skills that involve tracking sensations through mindful awareness, and using pendulation and breathing practice to rebalance the rhythms of your nervous system.

A foundational skill of this first stage is to learn how to work effectively with medical and other pain professionals. One way to begin this is by confronting four common myths about pain recovery. (Chapter 5 will offer further insight on working with professionals in the context of preparing for medical procedures.)

Debunking Your Myths about Recovery

When you are stalled in your pain recovery, the primary objective should be to develop strong alliances with treating professionals who are supportive and trustworthy. This is far from easy since you may have had negative experiences en route to reading this book. Yet often times it is not possible to recover from chronic pain by oneself. To get the help you want or need, it will be essential to learn how to work effectively with professionals.

One way of developing positive relationships is to clearly identify and then shift the negative beliefs you may have about recovering from pain. Your encounters with pain professionals can then become more productive and collaborative. Here are some common myths about recovering from pain that can spawn negative beliefs.

Myth 1: Nothing Can Help You with Your Pain

One of the most frequent self-limiting beliefs about pain treatment is the fear that nothing can help you with your pain. This often results in an unwillingness to take even small risks that might widen your window of tolerance or comfort zone, especially if it is initially painful.

As we've seen earlier, the anxiety or fear you may be carrying with you can trigger a pain trap: bracing in your body in response to fear, which creates more pain, leading to more fear, more bracing, and more pain and fear. This vicious cycle can contribute to a sense of feeling constantly vigilant. When a method does not seem to work, you may quickly spiral down into despair and hopelessness.

Is this already happening for you? If so, you may want to pause for a few moments and reflect on some recent sessions with members of your pain team to find out if the hard shell of anxious hypervigilance is preventing you from being open to what can begin to work for you.

The truth is that you need just one intervention that starts to work reliably to help you relieve and reverse your pain. It's best to use a multimodal approach, trying different methods and combinations of approaches until you discover a tool, or combination of tools, that brings about a significant positive effect. Then you'll need to work consistently with whatever basic approach holds the key to unlocking your pain, so that you are receiving reliable results over time.

Once a reliable source of relief is in place, even though your underlying pain problem might not be resolved, you may begin to experience a sense of control over your discomfort for the very first time. And once that happens, your body will support this shift by closing the pain gates and opening new positive pathways.[1]

Myth 2: A Magic Bullet Will Erase Your Pain

Another common myth is that there is a magic bullet to erase all of your pain. Individuals overwhelmed by pain understandably hope that they can find the one expert or technique to solve their pain. They hope that with just the right medication, newly minted procedure, surgery, or intervention that all their anguish will be over.

First of all, any expert, no matter how accomplished, can only be an expert on the methods they use. Only *you* can be an expert on your own pain. What functions best is a working partnership in which the professional and the person in pain truly collaborate—each does 50 percent of the work that needs to happen.

We firmly believe that there are sufficient technologies (biofeedback, TENS units, ASTYM, laser therapy, and so on) and methodologies (such as Pilates, Active Release Technique, network chiropractic, Feldenkrais, Alexander technique, homeopathic remedies, and supplements) to help every person into a manageable, regulated place with pain.[2] So it's just a question of finding which combination of approaches is going to do the job for you, who can best help you use these methods, and how long the process will take.

Myth 3: If you don't follow the directives you're given, you are not a good patient.

While it is necessary to give a particular treatment a chance to work, you are the only one who can ultimately determine whether that treatment is working for you. Professional help can be valuable to assess why a treatment method is not working for you, and to suggest what modifications might make it more effective.

We have seen many clients in pain make the error of holding on to an approach that is not working just to "prove" that they can make it work, or to show that they are doing everything possible to heal. This attitude can lead to a waste of energy when the time could be used to explore new possibilities. If you have doubt, it's usually best to request a consultation with your pain doctor or treating professional.

Myth 4: Pain medications create dependency and addiction, and won't help you recover.

Professionals, as well as patients, fear that pain medications can create dependency and addiction and don't help people really recover from pain.[3] Of course, there is some truth in this belief. Pain medications (when used for a prolonged time) can dampen an individual's felt sense. Because of this, overmedicated individuals cannot really connect enough to their bodies to find the resources that will help them resolve the underlying bracing, trauma, or blocked emotions that often maintain chronic pain conditions and inhibit healing.

For the majority of pain patients, however, medication at the right time and at the right dose can be lifesaving. For example, often short-term use of simple anti-inflammatory medication like ibuprofen can begin to reverse pain responses. This is extremely important because once inflammation rages out of control, it becomes increasingly difficult to break the pain cycle. Nipping serious pain in the bud, as soon as possible, is always better than waiting to see what happens. There are situations where anti-inflammatory medications, like ibuprofen, simply are not adequate. This is where narcotic and opioid medications can save the day. For example, when used for some days after surgery or after a serious injury to prevent "breakthrough" pain, these strong medications can be invaluable.

Rita, an otherwise very healthy ninety-three-year-old woman, began to have sudden nerve pain from the impingement of two thoracic disks; she began a serious downward spiral, despairing and saying bleakly, "My life is over." She experienced no pleasure in her usual daily activities. A simple recommendation made with the permission of Rita's doctor was that instead of taking only one ibuprofen per day (which was not enough for her level of inflammation and discomfort), she should increase her dosage to six to nine tablets per day. In two weeks, Rita's pain went from 9 on a 10-point pain scale to a 1or 2, and she was back to enjoying her life even though she was diagnosed with scoliosis and osteoporosis. This example illustrates the principle that changes which bring pain under control are much easier to sustain over time.

Many people stay away from medications because of their long-term effects, but in the short term, it is important to *get ahead of the pain and to stay ahead of the pain.* Most professionals now advocate this approach. But the problem for the person in pain is in knowing how to apply this principle in their pain situation. So while overmedication can be problematic, *under*-medication can be a problem as well.

Further Mastery of Body Awareness and Self-Regulation Skills

As we discussed earlier, in order to connect with body experience, it's important to learn how to bring awareness to body sensation—to the felt sense. In Peter's book *In an Unspoken Voice*, *embodiment* and *awareness* are described as "the twin sisters of mercy,"[4] because in addition to being essential for effective self-regulation of emotional and physical pain reactions, embodied awareness is a master tool for personal enrichment and self-discovery.

To experience embodied awareness, take notice of the underlying sensations that actually inform you about how you feel. If you were to be asked how you feel when you are stressed or in pain, a common answer might be, "I feel anxious" or "I feel upset." It's important to go further by becoming curious about *how you know* that you're feeling anxious or upset. Is there a tightness or burning that is happening right now inside of you that you are labeling "anxiety" or "upset"?

If this approach to discovery is not successful, we ask more specifically what kind of thoughts you might be having if you can't get to the body sensations. One common answer is expressed with a thought like: "I feel like I'm going to die; this is going to go on forever." Thoughts are interpretations and judgments of our feelings and sensations. We can't change our feelings and sensations with our thoughts, but our feelings can change our thoughts. The only way to change a feeling, however, is to let go of the thoughts, and focus on each particular feeling or sensation as it passes, or shifts to something new. So if you have a thought, you can simply affirm: "OK, I have the thought that I'm going to die and that this is going to go on forever." The next step could be to ask yourself, "What sensations in my body are associated with this thought?" Sometimes just naming thoughts and distinguishing them from sensations can lead to a positive shift into the felt sense.

It's also important to keep asking yourself direct questions about body experiences. This may lead to an internal exchange such as this one:

"How about my heart right now?"
"Yeah, it's beating fast."

"OK. So as I notice my heart beating fast, let's just notice
if it increases, or if it decreases, or if it remains the
same, or if I am becoming aware of something else."
"Oh, it's getting worse; it's getting worse, I don't want to
do this!"
"OK, it's getting worse, it's getting worse, and when it's
getting worse, what do I notice?"
"Well, that's interesting. It just started to slow down."

Often when you begin to focus on sensations like this, the feelings
will seem to get worse. But quickly after they worsen, they will begin
to change or even subside. This is the essence of self-regulation.
Focusing on one part of the "concept" being called "anxiety" is only
the starting point.

It's an interesting paradox that the more aware you become of
your *complete experience,* the less anxious and in pain you will feel.
Sometimes this shift comes from just naming the different elements of
the experience so that you create a secure container for what you are
experiencing. Sometimes this happens through increasing your range
of awareness, so that there is a shift into experiences that are neutral or
positive, or that evoke curiosity.

Expanding the Felt Sense

In chapter 2, we presented the exercise Exploring the Felt Sense (page
20). In the next exercise, we focus on how you might continue to further
develop your felt sense through embodied awareness.

EXERCISE: Developing the Felt Sense
🔊 Track 11

One way to learn to focus on sensation, especially if you tend to be
disconnected from your body, is through gentle tapping, not just on
certain parts of the body, but on the whole body, to gradually awaken

the felt sense of body experience. This kind of body tapping is different than tapping used to activate specific energy points. Avoid tapping on areas that are already painful or feel too vulnerable. Gently tap one hand with your other hand, then each arm, the shoulders, the neck, the head—just very gently tapping. This kind of tapping goes right into the sensory cortex. So again, gentle tapping without hurry, especially on the perimeter of the body, the legs, feet, arms, hands, and shoulders, can be helpful in restoring a body sense.[5]

Another basic body awareness technique is to squeeze your muscles gently. Do not squeeze your muscles to the point where it hurts. Cross your arms over your chest with your hands resting on your forearms. Then gently squeeze your arm muscles, squeeze the triceps and the biceps. Tell yourself, "These are my muscles; this is where I live." Again be careful of painful areas, but as you release the muscle, the discomfort may actually feel less than when you started.

If you'd like, describe your experiences with these tapping and squeezing techniques in your pain journal.

These body awareness exercises are two important and simple ways to develop the felt sense and help reduce dissociation. They can be used as a regular practice. Depending on your degree of dissociation, you may need to do these exercises every day and more than once during the day.

The same kinds of techniques can also help with the kind of pain that is caused by flooding (being overwhelmed). This situation refers to too much sensation as compared with the "nothingness" of dissociation or disconnection. One method to reduce flooding is to lie in a fetal position or other secure posture, while putting gentle pressure on your arm muscles or squeezing them gently. This can be very useful in deactivating and reducing the sense of overwhelm while increasing the ability to connect with your body.

The next time you are experiencing too much sensation, try this technique, and keep track of your experiences in your pain journal.

In order to make these changes, you need to learn to tolerate certain sensations of tingling, of vibration, of trembling, of heat and cold, and other sensory experiences that accompany the process of regulation. Whatever technique is used, the goal is to befriend your body sensations. And when you can do that, very often there can be a dramatic shift in your pain levels.

When starting any practice, it's important to understand that pain may become more acute for a short period of time. This is because if you've been either flooded or shut down and dissociated, there has been little possibility of really feeling your body experience. When it's possible to actually start feeling body responses, you may actually experience the pain more intensely at first. But generally, by practicing these kinds of self-regulatory felt-sense techniques, within a period of hours or a few days at most, the pain usually drops, and then you can become more aware of other sensations—the more pleasant ones. It is possible at this point to switch back and forth between the pleasant sensations and the painful sensations, so that you have another tool in this felt-sense shifting. You already know that your pain cycle can escalate. Now you can also discover how it can innately and progressively deescalate.

Dorothy: From Anxiety and Pain to Comfort and Balance

For five years, beginning soon after her father's death, Dorothy had struggled with terrible discomfort in her right abdominal area. She had undergone multiple intensive medical workups, including MRIs of the pain site, and many possible sources of her pain had been ruled out. There was no sign of muscle tearing, which was closest to Dorothy's own diagnosis, or bowel obstruction, diverticulitis, Crohn's disease, hernia, or GERD (gastroesophageal reflux disease). The possibility of cysts on the right ovary or on other nearby abdominal organs had also been dismissed through numerous examinations and tests.

During several meetings, Dorothy gently explored her right abdominal area. At first she had difficulty moving away from thoughts such as "I think it must be from when I moved all those boxes" and into sensations. Practice allowed her felt-sense awareness of her pain and fear to unfold in explorations like the following, where she was working with a therapist. (This inquiry could also be done with a friend, through a kind of inner dialogue, or a journaling practice.)

Dorothy: Now I'm aware of a pulsing.

Therapist: Can you show me through your hand and finger movement the speed and quality of that pulsing?

Dorothy: (Pauses.) As I'm moving my fingers, the rhythm reminds me of a trapped butterfly . . . and that's how I've been feeling, trapped. I'm trapped by this pain and have to organize my life around it—by not being able to eat what I enjoy, by not knowing when this terrible cramping will start again and force me to just lie down and do nothing. I will lose a day or two of my life on these occasions.

Therapist: Tell me how "trapped" feels right now in your body.

Dorothy: It's like a blockage. I stop breathing and moving. I stop doing anything because it hurts too much.

Therapist: And as you feel that blockage, what happens next in your body?

Dorothy: (Long pause.) Hmm. That's interesting. There's a little opening there . . . it's like a little trickle of energy is getting through. I'm afraid to feel it, though, because it's just going to disappear like so many times before. And that's even worse.

Therapist: Can you stay with the *sensation* of the tiny opening and its flow of energy as well as with your worry that it will disappear?

Dorothy: The opening seems stronger now. I don't know why. It's like it's answering my worry by saying, "I'm really here now. I'm not going away this time. I'm not going to leave you." (Dorothy begins sobbing.) That feels so good to hear.

Breathing and the Felt Sense

Continued use of basic breathing techniques is often the best way to extend and expand the felt sense. Most people are familiar with diaphragmatic breathing, so we usually start with some form of that practice. Whether you are flooded with pain or fear, or are more dissociated and disconnected, it will help to really feel your breath cycle. This next exercise will take you beyond the earlier exercise on modified diaphragmatic breathing (page 35) by incorporating the felt sense.

EXERCISE: Diaphragmatic Breathing and Felt Sense

To begin, bring your awareness to your diaphragm area just above your belly button. If it helps you to connect with your body, place one or both hands over this area. Practice following your breath until you feel a very basic connection with your breathing rhythms, with their tempo and consistency. Stay with your breathing until you feel comfortable that your next breath will come on its own. Feel the natural sense of expansion as your lungs and the muscles around your ribs expand when you breathe in, and then let go as you breathe out. Do you feel a difference in your felt sense of connection with your body?

Next, as you breathe in, allow yourself to become aware of the more expanded parts of the body and name them for yourself—for example: "an opening and movement of air from my belly up to my face and nose;" or "an expansion through my middle back and the sides of my body." When breathing out, focus on any constriction or discomfort you become aware of: "I notice tightness in my belly and a kind of collapse in my chest."

Practice using this technique consistently for a few days. What do you notice in general about your felt sense of your body? About your pain? Note your reactions to this exercise in your pain journal.

Another breathing technique to revisit is circle breathing, which was introduced in the exercise on page 24. Circle breathing is excellent preparation for the practice of pendulation, which we will explore later in this chapter, and also can stand alone as a self-regulation approach.

Sometimes it may be necessary to modify circle breathing further to find a better fit. For example, if you have asthma or other breathing problems, you may have trouble focusing on and staying with your breathing. It's often helpful in this case to take two or more breaths as part of the circle breathing practice, rather than just one breath as indicated in the earlier exercise. In this way, you can breathe up the more comfortable side of the body, and then breathe out and down the middle of your body, allowing your body to let go as you exhale. Then, with the second breath, breathe in through, and up, the middle of the body, and then breathe out down the less comfortable side.

We want to emphasize that there is no magic in any of these techniques. The positive effects are really all related to practice. The magic occurs when we allow the organism to use its native resilience to recover from pain. The simple techniques we've described are basic bridges from pain or numbness to body awareness, and ultimately to self-regulation and aliveness.

As always, if the technique you are practicing does not achieve the desired effect, stop your practice and move to another method until you find one that works for you.

The Role of Mindfulness, Connection, and Regulation

In chapter 3, we introduced mindfulness as an excellent way to observe body experience and you used mindful observation to practice securing a resting place in your body (page 31). In this chapter, we go further, introducing you to the scientific basis of mindfulness and linking this practice to the skills of embodiment and tracking.

As we practice mindfulness, we become aware of what we desire in life. We also learn how to focus on our intentions, particularly toward other people, to achieve those needs and desires. In a sense, we develop the attunement to know ourselves and our ambitions through attachment relationships with others. Individuals who've been impaired in their attachment experiences will frequently struggle with this process. So mindfulness practice is one way of beginning to repair some of the relationship issues and conflict within ourselves,[6] including those that originate from early childhood.

Psychiatrist Daniel Siegel has pointed out that circuits in our brains that are engaged while in a resting state appear to be related to the circuits that we use when we interact with other people. Thus, the social circuits of the brain that we use to understand the mind, feelings, intentions, and attitudes of others are similar to ones that we use to reflect on our own mind and body.[7]

The Mindful Brain

Siegel also points out that the prefrontal cortex is a brain structure almost entirely developed after birth through attachment or early bonding experiences with our parents and significant others. It is related to our later experience of a cohesive, whole self. Some of the functions of the prefrontal cortex include body regulation, attuned communication, affective or emotional balance, fear regulation, response flexibility, insight, empathy, and intuition.

In relationship to pain, the mindful brain can help us develop embodied awareness in three different ways. First, mindfulness can help us deal effectively with negative reactions that are related to stress, such as anxiety and anger, as well as dissociation and depression. Secondly, mindfulness can help us drop the habit of endlessly struggling and fighting against the pain, because it gives us a chance to pause and make other choices, which can lead to more pleasure and enjoyment in everyday life. Focusing on alternative decisions is another important skill for escaping the pain trap. As Albert Einstein once said: "The definition of insanity is doing the same thing again and again, and expecting a different result."

It's essential to understand how mindfulness also encompasses embodiment, or awareness of body sensation. It's far more than just awareness of the mind and its multiplicity of thoughts. The key to developing an effective pathway to self-regulation through mindfulness practice must also include the awareness of what we experience in our bodies.

The Importance of Mindful Embodiment

Mindfulness practice is an essential pathway to self-regulation through awareness of the "living, knowing" body. Our understanding of the process of healing is built upon the mind-body connection and also encompasses the mind-body-heart-spiritual/transpersonal connection. It's important for you to understand that the partnership between your mind and body (which of course is an artificial duality) involves using your mindful awareness to focus on the wisdom of the body, with the goal of really appreciating, understanding, and supporting that wisdom. The body and mind learn from each other. For example, when you become aware of just one single breath (see exercise on page 33), this can instantly create mind-body partnership, because you're bringing mindful awareness to your body experience within the powerful, accessible container of one breath cycle.

Tracking Specific Sensations

As you've been learning throughout this program, felt-sense awareness is the conduit within which we experience the totality of sensation. Every experiential event, including pain, can be experienced first through its separate components, and eventually as a unified whole. The felt sense includes, of course, the external physical senses, such as sight (images), sounds, smells, and tastes, but also includes important data from our internal awareness of the body—including its movements, temperature, postures, gestures, and even tensions, as well as expansions. Emotions such as sadness, fear, disgust, joy, and anger also influence the felt sense. The felt sense is ever changing and typically more vague, more complex, and more dynamic than emotions, however, and is the larger landscape on which our emotions roam.

Learning to track specific sensations will help you further regulate your pain reliably, through work with pain triggers, and give you further skills in order to work effectively with pendulation, the premier integrative tool for self-regulation.

Neuroscience suggests that emotional and physical pain involve the same parts of the brain. For this reason, we can assume that physical and emotional pain influence and feed off of each other. This next practice exercise will help you better understand some of the interactions between your physical and emotional pain.

EXERCISE: Interrupting Pain Triggers
🔊)) Track 12

Focus on an emotional trigger related to your pain condition. This can be a current situation or a past memory that stirs up anger, fear, grief, or other strong emotions. Your reaction should be within a *moderate* range; that is, don't choose something that you know will be overwhelming. Perhaps this was a message given to you by a doctor, a reaction of a friend or loved one to your pain limitations, or an emotional injury of rejection or hurt.

Slowly scan your entire body to find the location where the sensation resides most intensely. Is it in your chest, your abdomen, or someplace else? Focus all of your attention on this area and direct your breath to the center of it. Experience and name the physical sensations that you find while continuing to breathe into this area. What do you notice as you continue this process?

If you become uncomfortable, redirect your sensory awareness to positive memories that are calming and balancing, such as a conflict-free experience (see page 42). Then practice shifting back and forth between the positive sensations and those of the emotional pain trigger you explored.

What happens? Does your reaction to the pain trigger diminish? Please note your experience in your pain journal.

The Promise of Pendulation

You may be wondering, "How can such simple practices as embodied awareness and breathing really shift *my* pain?" After all, you've tried so many other things, how can you be sure that what we're suggesting really works?

These are fair questions given the magnitude of the usual struggles with persistent and chronic pain. The answer lies in the innate power of rhythm. The energy-level rhythms of the nervous system, at its most primitive reptilian-level, oscillate naturally like a pendulum. For example, we breathe in—we breathe out. We are active and alert—we are tired and go to sleep and rest. We contract—we expand. This is the basic rhythm pattern of life.

The tool of pendulation is a simple, powerful way to harness and shift these rhythms so that the nervous system rebalances from the toll of pain, stress, and trauma. Simply put, pendulation is one of the few basic tools that can intervene effectively and reliably with hyperarousal, with the freeze response, and with difficult emotions in general.

There are many methods that can be used to intervene with the fight and the anger end of the spectrum, as well as with the flight and fear end. Modalities for pain treatment, including psychotherapy and body therapies, are overflowing with many possible approaches. Yet there are almost none that are available for direct intercession with the freeze response. And since many, if not all, individuals who have been in pain for any length of time are blocked from moving out of pain by unresolved and unreleased freeze reactions, it's easy to understand why this route to healing *must* be addressed.

Most experts now agree that the hallmark of trauma is being frozen, stuck, or trapped in fear, helpless collapse, dissociation, terror, and rage. Pendulation allows you to go indirectly to the edges of where you are stuck, and to begin to move through and out of freeze and immobility so that you have access again to your action systems. It can then help you to access the more active defenses of fight and flight.

We have found that working from the most primitive body level upward toward feelings, thoughts, and perceptions provides the most efficient and effective pathway for lasting healing. This "bottom up" processing, assisted by the practice of pendulation, is the crucial tool for the reliable resolution of pain and trauma symptoms.

Pendulation helps us rock gently back and forth between contraction and expansion, between fear and safety, between anger and calm, between grief and acceptance, and between inaction and action. Through this practice, many people can be helped to shift out of pain and onto tiny islands of relative comfort and positive connection in a very short time. It is vital for any person in pain to practice and get to know intimately the rhythms of pendulation. This practice will teach you the dynamics of balance and certain change, the gentle predictability of knowing that, no matter how excruciating your pain is in this moment, in the very next one, your experience can and will shift.

You have already been preparing for pendulation by working with circle breathing and other practices presented so far in this program. Even if you have practiced pendulation many times before, we encourage you to try the following exercise to further refine your skills and your understanding of this vital process.

EXERCISE: Pendulation and the Rhythms of Pain
🔊)) Track 13

Find a position where you can sit comfortably or lie down with the right type of support that allows you to be alert and relaxed without falling asleep. Make sure you can be free from distractions for about fifteen minutes.

1. Begin by exploring your body experience. Scan your body for areas of openness and expansion, as well as those of contraction or tightness. Using your ability to connect with your felt sense, find the smallest areas of expansion as well as the largest; identify the same parameters for tightness, constriction, or pain.

2. Imagine that you are going on an expedition of discovery. Explore each island of comfort or expansion and each area of constriction as if you could pull up a chair next to it and just observe it. What sensations do you find? Use your breath to explore more deeply by sending it into the center of each location. What else do you encounter?

3. Now use your focused attention to shift back and forth from the smallest area of discomfort to the smallest area of comfort, bridging back and forth several times. Feel the sense of shifting from constriction to expansion. Do you feel a sense of gradually encountering a little more expansion each time? If not, what differences do you experience?

4. Gradually shift your attention to the medium-sized areas of constriction and expansion. Feel the rhythm of bridging back and forth, back and forth. What happens this time?

5. Finally, travel from the largest area of discomfort or pain to the largest area of expansion or comfort. Again, shift back and forth several times using your breath to occupy fully each location. Notice the

rhythm of this movement. Does it feel different from the earlier bridging? If so, how?

6. How does the sense of flow and expansion help to shift specific areas of pain and tightness? What is the general, overall change in the sensations of constriction that you started with? What does this teach you about the overall rhythms of pain?

With practice, pendulation can help restore resilience obstructed by pain. Instead of feeling beaten down by hopelessness and despair, you can discover the vibrant promise of change in each moment. Because you are pacing yourself, you follow your own natural, innate rhythms, slowing down when the experience of shifting back and forth feels overwhelming and perhaps going a little faster and deeper or shifting back and forth more times when you feel more disconnected.

Because pendulum rhythms help us to find balance between pleasant and unpleasant sensations, we can trust our bodies more deeply and accept where somatic experience leads us, especially since we have learned again and again that our destination can shift in the next moments. Gradually, we reach acceptance, knowing that even if we feel terrible, that feeling can and will change. This understanding releases us from the pervasive sense of doom that persistent pain often creates.

STAGE 2: ONGOING TRANSFORMATION

Once you create a platform of greater confidence in self-regulating your pain, built on the predictable rhythms that pendulation can create, the next stage of recovery from pain is ongoing transformation. You will be able to build securely on the pendulum platform, using numerous tools and experiences. This can be a rich passage of discovery and migration back to wholeness.

The Force of Spirituality

When people in pain learn to shift from the avoidance of body experience in order to avoid the hurt of pain, they begin to trust and befriend the wisdom of the body. During this time, you can continue to build trust, strength, and resilience as you create more and more experiences of embodied self-awareness. This path will help you reclaim your body from the ravages of pain by finding and following body sensations, feeling the rhythms of change, and using your own touch as well as receiving touch (from a massage therapist, for example) in order to amplify and deepen that basic connection between mind and body. As these connections deepen, another healing dimension, the force of spirituality, will naturally emerge.

The connection between pain, trauma, and spirituality is an important one. Over many years of practice, we have been privileged to witness profound and authentic transformations during the process of healing with many clients. As these individuals have mastered the traumas that have haunted them emotionally, physically, and psychologically, amazing surprise benefits occur, including the release from pain and the opening to joy, exquisite clarity, effortless focus, and sometimes an all-embracing sense of peace and oneness. In addition, many of these individuals describe deep and abiding experiences of wholeness and compassion, especially self-compassion.

We want you to know that it's possible to develop an alchemical type of relationship, a transmuting relationship, between pain areas and pleasurable areas, between open areas and constricted areas. It's not that pain is bad, and pleasure is good. What's important is the *balance* between pain and pleasure and being able to shift between them. As you engage in this seemingly magical/mystical process, the two polarities of pleasure and pain no longer exist as polarities; instead, they are integrated into a new dynamic synthesis.

Interestingly, when people are moving through a true healing process, they almost won't notice that a pain or symptom has abated or even gone away. Sometimes weeks after healing work, they'll say, "You know, this is strange, I came in here because of my chronic lower-back pain, and I just realized that I don't have it anymore. It has just faded into the background." Sometimes, when we don't ask our clients about their pain symptoms for a short while, we are then gratified to discover that these difficulties have mysteriously vanished.

How can we explain these shifts? Often they come through spiritual experiences. If you have trouble with the term "spirituality" because of its association with religious doctrine, then you might think of these experiences as strong positive conflict-free feelings that are critical in the self-healing process and to the self-regulatory process. The experience of joy for many pain patients is one of the important pleasures they feel robbed of. Introducing mindfulness or other approaches, such as gratefulness, as pathways to rediscovering joy in your life can be very important.

The Practice of Gratitude

One of the best ways we know to expand joy as well as acceptance and compassion for yourself is through the practice of gratitude. Of course, when you're in pain, this is highly challenging because you might not sense there are many things for which you can actively feel grateful.

Brother David Steindl-Rast, Benedictine monk and well-known speaker on gratefulness as spiritual practice, teaches that there is a direct link between joy and gratefulness.[8]

Rather than experiences of joy creating gratefulness, as most people believe, Brother David believes that when we are grateful, our gratitude is what leads us into joy. He defines gratefulness as full appreciation for something that is freely given, beginning with the gift of life itself. So rather than waiting until we are joyful to feel grateful, he recommends that we cultivate daily gratitude, since the more grateful we feel, the more likely it is that we will find joy in our lives. This view is also seen in many forms of Buddhism.

Brother David suggests that we practice finding one thing each day for which we are grateful. This gift should be something we have never before focused on with a heart of gratitude. If you are interested in this process, follow this practice for a week and record the results in your pain journal. What changes for you? Does this practice make a difference in your daily experience?

According to the Institute of HeartMath, gratefulness and appreciation for self and others are among the most concrete and easiest positive feelings to self-generate in order to shift out of stressful, painful emotions. HeartMath research has shown that people who use simple tools for this purpose experience lasting benefits, including increased physical health and emotional well-being resulting in pervasive re-patterning.

The HeartMath program is designed to help people develop empowering, heart-based living. The focus is on developing positive intentions and actions in daily life originating from the intuitive wisdom of our hearts that takes the form of sincere appreciation, caring, and kindness toward self and others. HeartMath tools are based on twenty years of careful research on factors such as the impact of stress on heart rate variability and the benefits of aligning physical, mental, emotional, and spiritual dimensions of experience.[9]

HeartMath methods emphasize a two-way energy exchange between heart and brain. Stressful emotions, such as fear, anger, and grief, make our heart rhythms more erratic, while positive emotions produce *heart coherence,* a regulated, fluid pattern of heart waves, which is linked to lower stress, higher energy levels, and the synchronization of the cranial brain and the "heart brain." The practice of heart-centered gratitude, for example, can increase measures of heart coherence. If you'd like to practice a simple HeartMath technique, try this mini-exercise:[10]

> *First focus* your attention in the area of your heart, much like you would focus on your right elbow, left foot,

or both ears. If helpful, place one or both hands over your heart to support this connection.

Imagine that your breath is flowing in and out through your chest where you sense your heart's location. Breathe in gently and steadily through your heart and out through your heart for about the same duration of time. Repeat until your breathing feels slow and easy.

Continue breathing in and out through your heart. Think of a positive feeling of appreciation for someone you know, a pet, or a place in nature. Keep breathing in and out through your heart while focusing on this source of appreciation. (Note: it is not necessary to actually *feel* appreciation.)

What changes do you notice? If you'd like, expand your practice of pendulation from earlier in this chapter (page 69) by focusing first on sensations related to emotional or physical pain or discomfort. Then shift to your sense of heart-centered gratitude breathing, which you just practiced. Let yourself shift back and forth for a few cycles. How does your breathing change? How do the sensations related to emotional or physical pain change?

Self-Love and Compassion

Generally, to enhance the spiritual dimension of experience, we think it's important to look at your intentions toward yourself. There are many ways that you can develop self-love and compassion, whether or not you consider this spiritual practice. People in pain have an especially difficult time loving themselves because their pain crowds out pleasure and balance from their lives. They are also challenged because they feel profound helplessness about being able to regulate pain in a positive direction.

One simple way to access a spiritual focus is to become aware of your positive intentions toward yourself, even saying the words out loud to see if you can find resonance with those words in your body as part of the felt sense. Reminding yourself, "I want to love myself," is every bit as important as any technique you might use to manage a particular kind of pain.

Another pathway to help you develop self-love is to focus on self-compassion. Although there are many methods that can help you find and strengthen compassion for yourself, the practice of lovingkindness (*metta*) meditation is one that many people find helpful.

To try this mini-exercise, sit in a comfortable, upright position. Close your eyes if you wish and take three slow, easy breaths from your heart as well as your diaphragm. If helpful, place one hand in each location.

Form an image of yourself just as you are, whether sitting or lying down. View and sense your posture and whatever body sensations you are aware of. Focus on the thought that every living being wants to live peacefully and happily. Connect with your own deep wish for this: "Just as all beings want to be happy and free from suffering, may I be happy and free from suffering." Pause and feel the warmth of that loving intention.

Keeping in mind the image of yourself as you are right now and feeling goodwill in your heart, repeat any or all of the following statements:

- May I be safe.
- May I be healthy.
- May I be free of suffering.
- May I live with grace and ease.

Pause to feel each phrase in your body. Repeat each one you choose a few times to connect fully with the positive intention. Sometimes it is helpful to repeat just one word, such as "safe, safe, safe," to fully experience the meaning.

If you become distracted, refocus on your image or sense of yourself in your current body position, and place one hand on your heart and one on your diaphragm, breathing easily and freely for two to three breaths. Then, return to the phrases. Remember that distractions will *always* arise and that your intention is to bring love to yourself. Sitting with yourself in this practice can be like sitting with a dear friend who is not feeling well. You cannot cure what is wrong with your friend but you can offer the kindness that is deserved. [11]

When this experience feels complete, open your eyes and write for a few minutes about your experiences in your pain journal.

Transforming Persistent Pain Patterns

We might ask someone who is struggling with seemingly unpredictable pain spikes: "What are the steps that lead up to the negative result?" That is, what precedes the unwanted condition of lying in bed feeling hopeless or struggling with panic for hours on end? The purpose of the question is to explore how you can intervene *before* you end up in that unacceptable place.

Once you have determined the sequence in your "chain of pain," it is much easier to shift toward comfort and wholeness by shifting one link in the chain. Much like the way a mobile works, if you touch or change one element, the entire structure of the pain pattern often changes.

The easiest way to start is to become curious or mindful about the chain of events that leads to a pain spike, rather than suppressing or trying to control it. You might want to keep a record of times when your pain suddenly increases. Practice mindfulness to determine the sequence of behaviors, thoughts, emotional feelings, and sensorimotor sensations that might be contributing to a particular type of symptom.

EXERCISE: A New Approach to Journaling
◀)) Track 14

Many pain patients have been asked to keep pain journals by their treating professionals, and often the patients' perceptions are that this practice does not lead to any significant changes. Principles of brain plasticity suggest that we are motivated by novelty,[12] so if an assignment does not challenge you to extend beyond what has been learned previously, it may be difficult to stay motivated.

One way to get creative, and thereby motivated, with this journaling practice is to work backward. Think about the last time your pain spiked unexpectedly and you collapsed into it. Maybe you crawled into bed because you were giving up. Maybe you decided you didn't want to live with the level of pain you were feeling. The important question is, what were you seeing, feeling, and thinking just *before* you decided to get into bed, or whatever intolerable state you collapsed into?

Then ask yourself, "What happened before that?" Take a few minutes to write down your observations of the sequence, and continue going back in time as you become more aware of the whole sequence. Work backward, from the peak of pain and collapse, moving closer and closer to the precipitating event(s), and to the first link in the chain that you can identify. Try to name each chunk or link in the chain that led up to your pain spike.

As you think now about this sequence, what could you change with the least amount of effort? For example, you might track back to the desire to go for a walk and then realize you had the *thought* that walking might cause more pain . . . then you felt a knot in your gut and a tensing of your neck and shoulders . . . this tension then caused the pain to jump from a 3 to a 6. Perhaps, by becoming aware of the thought, you could decide to take a short, easy walk and then increase the distance only if the pain did not actually go up. Or by noticing the tension you might use one of the breathing exercises to reduce the tension before it led to the increased pain.

It's important to leave this process open-ended. Even small bits of new information can be gained from thoughts, sensations, emotions, images, or movements that may have been previously dissociated. This can be an effective method that leads to pattern interruption and change. Sometimes all you need to do, in order to shift the outcome, is to change one component of the sequence as we just illustrated.

Keep a record of where this experience leads you. Make sure to journal about each step toward success. ✐

Resolving Barriers to Recovery

We invite you to consider further how you can identify and remove barriers that may be contributing to persistent pain and blocking your ongoing transformation process. Here are some common barriers we see in pain treatment that is not going well.

Focusing on Pathology Instead of Skills

Many individuals struggling with pain have been undermined or disparaged in different ways by professionals who have misdiagnosed or mislabeled them, focusing only on pathology and saying, "This is what you're doing wrong" or "This is what you aren't doing well enough." Instead, we focus on prescriptions like the following: "You can learn a set of skills, so that you can begin shifting the patterns of your pain, whether it's through Somatic Experiencing, breathing, imagery, or other combinations of methods. Once you have experienced even a small difference in your relationship with pain, then everything will be different."

Struggling with Accepting the Pace of Your Recovery

You may be aware of thoughts like, "I should be in a different place by now" or "I've already learned breathing techniques and I don't think they're going to help me." It's important to know that in every single moment where you can bring awareness to your body there is the potential of change. Every moment! That means there are always opportunities for a miracle to take place.

Fearing That the Old Pain Patterns Will Return

Another frequent block occurs when longstanding pain sufferers start to feel better, and then immediately begin to fear that the old pain patterns will come back. It's important to accept that these patterns may well return, but with the understanding that this *is* the nature of recovery; pain comes and goes while we stay focused on resolving the underlying pattern.

This is also the way that our human organism integrates change. Toddlers don't just get out of bed one day and start walking across the floor. We have to learn gradually, by trial and error, or through experiment and discovery, what works—what supports us, and what doesn't. Creating a pragmatic treatment situation that supports people to develop curiosity about what is going to work, rather than what *should* work, is essential.

"I Can't Imagine Being Without Pain"

While this may sound silly, a fourth obstacle is not knowing what to do without the pain. You may have become so used to pain that your whole life is organized around avoiding the situations and people that you have found to be triggering. When the pain dissolves, a near panic may arise. Questions such as: "What's going to happen now? What am I going to do with my life?" start popping up. The fear of not knowing how to re-engage in life, be with people, and become more active, can be overwhelming. So it's important to give yourself time to adjust to being without pain, since pain has become so familiar, and the familiarity becomes your friend. Pain often becomes a way to avoid dealing with things (including feelings) that frighten us. Sometimes people even feel a kind of sadness about being without pain, like the loss of an important relationship.

Struggling with Attachment Issues

Yet another issue that can interfere with forward progress is the role of attachment. This refers to the early bonding between our infant and/or child selves, and our first caregivers. Many people who have had problematic pain conditions also had disturbed early bonding experiences. Either they have experienced benign neglect, or, in some cases, have had relational experiences that were very intrusive, negative, and abusive.

Attachment issues can often skew our perceptions of, and relationships with, treating professionals. Sometimes pain sufferers can perceive their doctor as an infallible god-like being who always knows what's best. On the other hand, the doctor might be perceived as an unfeeling, distant authoritarian figure who doesn't care about your needs. Neither of these perceptions is necessarily accurate, and acting as if either one is true can be very counterproductive.

When you enter into pain treatment, it is essential that you form a collaborative relationship with your treating professional. What this means is that you will want to learn to give your input, ask questions, and advocate for your right to have as much choice as possible. (We will discuss this more in chapter 5.)

If you experience a power struggle with your pain professional, this is not unusual. It may help to recognize some of the common signs of power struggles:

- the feeling that you are not understood or listened to
- a sense that you and your ideas are being dismissed or devalued
- the belief that your goals are not respected and that the professional "presumes he or she knows what's best for you"

Develop a Pain Plan

It is important to create a pain plan with your surgeon, physician, physical therapist, chiropractor, or any other health professional who will be helping to treat and monitor your pain. If a pain plan with clear goals is not in place, it will be difficult to evaluate your progress and move forward in the most efficient and effective ways possible. (See Zina's pain plan, on page 133.)

Outside a group practice or rehab facility, it can be challenging to create a pain team with a variety of practitioners. So when you require additional treatment services, ask the treating professionals with whom you already have a good relationship for referrals. This will ensure that your treatment is as cohesive as possible and that your providers will exchange information and consult with each other.

Pacing

A final note on the journey back from pain and the pilgrimage of ongoing transformation relates to the issue of pacing. Regardless of the method or technique you're using, it's important to pace your interventions with pain. If the pace you are using is fear-based (for example, influenced by the fear that you're not doing enough or the fear that you'll never get better, and so on), you will end up feeling overwhelmed.

It's important to titrate, or naturally dilute, your exposure to the trauma of pain and the pain of trauma by approaching both aspects carefully, in small bits that will be less likely to overwhelm you. Titration means that, though you may reach your goals more slowly, you will more likely sustain forward progress without becoming destabilized or having setbacks. If you are struggling with a pace that is slower than you would like, ask yourself questions like the following:

- Has my pain significantly improved in the last six months?
- Am I moving steadily forward even if I am taking small steps?
- If I stay on the path I'm on now with my pain, will I be likely to make the changes I want to make?

It is much more important to perceive the positive trends in your recovery than to become obsessive about your progress. We will discuss this issue further in later chapters.

CHAPTER FIVE

Working with Specific Pain Conditions

BEFORE WORKING WITH SPECIFIC PAIN CONDITIONS, it is essential to review all your medical assessments and previous treatment experiences. It is good to know the history of your pain condition, any diagnoses you have received, and also how you understand these labels. In addition, it is important to know what treatments you have experienced and how successful these have been, as well as what types of professionals you have worked with. We suggest that you review this information for yourself and write it down—that way your current doctor has all of your information on hand so that she or he can best help you. This is the beginning of forming a working alliance that will maximize positive results.

We must always be open to the possibility that there can be structural or organic causes of pain. It's essential to explore such "hard wiring" sources even though there may also be evidence of psychological components such as abuse or loss. It is always necessary to consider *both* physical factors and psychological/emotional/traumatic factors when deciding how to begin dealing with specific pain syndromes.

Ask yourself how much of the pain that you are experiencing now is related to your medical diagnosis? If the answer is, "I think it's 100 percent related to what the doctor told me," then you should focus more closely on reviewing our tips and guidance about getting the medical help you need. But if the answer is, "I feel like I've done a lot of healing. And yet, I think I still have a lot of stress that comes from the accident (or whatever event generated the pain in the first place)," then most certainly begin to look for possible emotional and traumatic sources. Likewise, if there seem to be earlier traumatic experiences that have not been resolved, this too might indicate a contributing factor to ongoing psychological stress/pain and prompt you to investigate further.

We begin by focusing on one of these two sides, either structural or "psychological," to keep things simple. But we never neglect the other. So for example, even though there might be physical injury, this does not eliminate the need to work on the traumatic and emotional aspects. We also encourage you, when working on these emotional aspects of your pain, not to eliminate the possibility that there might also be a mechanical issue at hand, such as something being torn, ruptured, or broken. But at the same time, you don't want to search endlessly for an organic cause when it simply might not exist. Also, it's important to consider the fact that for some people, getting a specific pain diagnosis can be more stressful than enlightening, especially if the pain is related to a life-threatening condition like cancer.

When working with any specific pain condition, we consider five levels of trauma. You will notice our references to these trauma dimensions throughout this chapter and elsewhere in this program.

1. *Trauma that is directly linked causally to the pain.*
   Some key examples are in the aftermath of illnesses, accidents, injuries, and surgeries.

2. *Single event trauma that precedes the pain.*
   This can include falls and other accidents (as in #1), but more broadly involves events like rape, robbery, mugging, and natural disasters.

3. *Developmental trauma.*
   This includes prenatal, perinatal, and postnatal distress, as well as issues with early parental bonding and ongoing parental relationships. This "attachment trauma" is different from single event trauma because it is generally pervasive and unconscious. Sometimes, if the child or mother is ill, bonding is interfered with. This can be particularly problematic if the mother suffers from postpartum depression. This kind of early trauma can lay a foundation for later pain conditions. If your parents are still alive, they might possibly provide some information. Of course this can be tricky, though sometimes a frank discussion can, in itself, be healing.

4. *Childhood abuse.*
   Molestation, neglect, loss, and other kinds of repetitive emotional and psychological trauma frequently result in dissociation and can be the most corrosive roots of pain because they are often caused by the individuals who are supposed to love and protect us. These kinds of confusing situations make it very difficult to feel anger and so we often turn it on ourselves. Both abuse and developmental arrests can slow down the recovery from pain. If you suffer from the effects of these issues, patience and persistence are important comrades on your journey.

5. *Trauma caused by chronic pain conditions.*
   Any chronic pain condition that has persisted can
   become traumatizing in and of itself. Pain causes fear
   and contributes to the emotional pain of depression.
   Each person's specific pain condition has unique
   undermining effects on mind, body, heart, spirit, and
   on daily life functioning.

Even if you do not suffer from the particular pain conditions described
in this chapter, you can still benefit from reading about each condition
and the methods used to cope with and possibly transform it. We have
organized this material as a general progression from relatively simple to
deeper and more complex pain syndromes. Therefore, we will start with
the more common neck and back pain problems.

CHRONIC NECK, BACK, AND SHOULDER PAIN

When this kind of pain is in the acute phase, it is easily treated by rest,
cold, and anti-inflammatory medications and often goes away on its
own. However, when this type of condition becomes chronic, the situation becomes more elusive because the causes may not be easy to trace
to a precipitating event. Diagnosis can be a lengthy process and this
may mean that it takes the patient longer to find relief. The assessment
might include MRIs, CT scans, and X-rays, various painful injections
including epidurals, nerve root blocks, joint injections, and other types
of nerve function evaluations. Of course, it is best if diagnosis can be
done with non-invasive, non-painful procedures. This is something to
consider with your physician or medical team.

Possible causes of back pain can include simple "muscle strains,"
structural issues like disc problems that include sciatica, joint pain,
and stenosis (narrowing of the spinal channel due to arthritis); and
structural irregularities including scoliosis and osteoporosis. Still other

sources of serious pain can include tumors, infections, and neurological problems.

The shoulders are one of the most common regions of pain problems and are particularly distressing because they are the most movable joints in the body and are used repeatedly for so many necessary movements. Causes of shoulder pain can include rotator cuff problems, tears and tendonitis, ligaments that tighten and cause "frozen" shoulder, and injuries that can fracture or separate the shoulder.

Vince: A Frozen Shoulder

Vince's symptoms had begun a few months before our appointment. He was working in his garage and picked up a starter motor to put into his car. As he lifted it, he felt "a twinge of something in his arm." The next day his shoulder felt tight and sore. Over time, the pain became more acute and his range of motion progressively worsened, becoming chronic.

Vince's story is surprisingly common: when the amount of pain isn't congruent with the circumstances of a minor accident, we then begin to explore a possible trauma-related reason behind it.

Not surprisingly, Vince attributed his shoulder "strain" to working on his car. This is somewhat like the person who reaches down and picks up a piece of paper, only to have their back go into spasm. Common sense, and the clinical observation of most chiropractors, physical therapists, and massage therapists, dictates that this was already "back primed"—an accident waiting to happen. In Vince's case, since there was no apparent physical injury, his physical therapist referred him to me in the hope of avoiding more difficult procedures.

Vince was obviously confused about seeing a "mind doctor," and was reluctant to engage with me. Sensing this, I reassured him that I would not be asking him personal questions, but would just focus on helping him get rid of his symptoms. "Yeah," he said, "my body sure is broke." I asked him to show me how far he could move his arm *before* it started to hurt. He moved it a few inches and then looked up at me: "That's about it." "OK, now I want you to move it the same way, but *much* slower, like this." I showed him with my arm. "Huh," he replied as he glanced at his arm. He was clearly surprised that he could move it a few inches further without the pain. "Even slower, this time, Vince. Let's see what happens this time . . . I want you to really give it your *full attention;* focus your mind on your arm now." Moving slowly allowed him a greater awareness of his arm. Just moving it quickly, without mindfulness, would have been likely to recreate the protective holding pattern, causing more pain.

His hand began to tremble and Vince looked to me for reassurance. "Yes, Vince, just let that happen . . . it's a good thing . . . it's your muscles starting to let go. Try to keep your mind focused there, with your arm and with the trembling . . . just let your arm move the way it wants to." The trembling went on for a while and then stopped; his forehead broke out in sweat.

As he moved to the edge of the bracing pattern, some of the energy held in his muscular-defense pattern began to release. This included the involuntary, autonomic nervous system reactions, such as shaking, trembling, sweating, and temperature changes. Because these are sub-cortical actions, the person does not have a feeling of control over his or her reactions. This may be quite unsettling at first. My function here was that of a coach/midwife, helping him to befriend these alien sensations, especially since he was wholly unaccustomed to involuntary reactions that he couldn't control.

"What is this, why is it happening?" he asked me in the voice of a frightened child. "Vince, I'm going to ask you to just close your eyes for a minute now and go inside your body . . . I'll be right here." After some moments of silence, his hands and arm began to extend outward: his whole arm, shoulders, and hands were now shaking more intensely. "It's OK for that to happen," I encouraged him, "Just let it do what it needs to do and keep feeling your body."

"It feels cold then hot," he said as he continued to reach out, moving now to about 45 degrees. Then he halted abruptly. His eyes opened wide, amazed that he could reach out so far without pain. At the same time, he seemed agitated; his face suddenly turned pale. He complained of feeling sick.

Instead of backing off, I coached him to stay present with his physical sensations. He started to breathe rapidly. "Oh my God, I know what this is." "Yes, good," I interrupted, "but let's just stay with the sensations for a little longer, then we'll talk about it, if you want. Is that OK?" Vince nodded and moved his arm back and forth from his shoulder as though he were sawing a piece of wood in slow motion. The trembling increased and decreased again, then settled. Tears flowed freely from his eyes. He took a deep spontaneous breath and then reached out, fully, in front of himself. "It doesn't hurt at all!" This corresponds with what we often have found with chronic pain: there is generally an underlying bracing pattern, and when the bracing pattern resolves, the pain often dissolves.

Working with Bracing Patterns

A large percentage of chronic neck, shoulder, and back pain is related to accident and injury. Our musculoskeletal system is designed to protect our bodies from threat of harm by bracing. Pain problems occur when these bracing patterns are never released. For Vince, it was the slow mindful movements that let him resolve his bracing pattern. Although Vince's body had already developed this bracing pattern, it took the minor strain from lifting the starter motor into his car to catalyze the reaction that set off the pain.

Vince Discovers What Emotions Were Locked in His Shoulder

At the end of his session, Vince opened his eyes and looked at me. Because of the connections made between his mind awareness and his body sensations, he was now able to form new meanings. He told me about the following event. About eight months earlier, he had gone shopping for his wife. As he came out of the grocery store, he heard a loud crash. Across the street, a car had smashed into a light pole. He dropped his shopping bag and ran to the accident. The driver, a woman, sat motionless in an apparent state of shock. The motor of the car was still running so he reached across her inert body to turn off the key, which is standard procedure to prevent fires or explosion. Just as he started to turn the key, he saw a young child in the passenger seat, his head fatally injured by an air bag. And then Vince told me *why* his shoulder got frozen: "I was fine before I saw the kid. As a fireman, I'm used to doing things like that, things that are dangerous . . . but when I saw the kid, part of me wanted to grab my arm back and turn away . . . I felt like puking . . . and the other part just stayed there and did what I had to do . . . sometimes it's really hard to do what you have to do." I agreed. "Yes, it's hard and you and your buddies keep doing it anyway. Thank you."

"Hmm," he added as he was leaving, "I guess I have to learn to mind my body." Vince had learned that mind and body are not separate entities; that he was a whole person. He said he wanted to learn more about himself and came in for three more sessions. He learned how to better handle stressful and conflicting situations and, needless to say, didn't need surgery.

While it was Vince's shoulder that was frozen, any part of our bodies can become frozen. By gently teasing out the conflicting forces and letting each one have its unobstructed voice, we too can thaw our frozen parts (one to reach out—and the other to retract in horror, in Vince's case). In the slow mindful movement of sawing his hand back and forth, Vince began to explore the inner movement "held in check" and locked into a bracing pattern. He had now separated two conflicting impulses: one involving reaching toward the keys and the other of pulling away in revulsion.

Bill

Another example is Bill, the patient with shoulder pain in chapter 1 who was able to resolve his pain by being supported gently, and gradually releasing his arm and its attachments through the mid-back area.

With help, he first tracked the bracing patterns to his fall into the water during the weekend celebration of his engagement as a young man, and later realized that these patterns overlapped with his headlong bicycle-crash into the utilities truck. As his arm and shoulder were cradled, Bill experienced gentle waves of trembling and shaking, which allowed the constriction to release. Over the span of several sessions, the neuromuscular pain, which had been locked in his body for more than six years, was released and resolved.

Now, while these cases are quite dramatic, you can certainly learn to work with various types of shoulder, neck, and back pain using the exercises in this book, including the following exercise.

Possibilities for Working with Locked Neck, Back, and Shoulder Pain

If you have problems in these (or other) areas of your body, take a few minutes to try a simple experiment, applying some of the principles that worked for Vince and Bill.

Sense the location that feels locked or constricted. Explore the sensations in the area surrounding the locked place. Name these for yourself using the language of sensation: tight, constricted, cold, hot, tingly, vibrating, shaking, trembling, and so forth.

Begin to shift your breathing so you can begin to explore the locked area. Imagine that you can breathe into the center of the locked area. Notice what begins to happen. Is there expansion? How do you know?

Sense any movement your body might want to make. Imagine the movement before you allow it to begin. Like Bill, does your arm want to be supported and

cradled with pillows or a soft blanket so that it can
gently vibrate or tremble to release the shock of a
current or past injury? Like Vince, does your arm want
to reach out in front of you to make rhythmic motions?

Slowly, and with gently directed awareness, allow these
movements to begin. As you sense the motions, allow
them to continue more slowly still. You might inhale
as you allow part of a movement, and as you exhale,
pause and feel your body's response. Continue until
you reach a sense of completion, at least for now.

If you'd like, spend a few minutes recording your experience in your pain
journal. Over time, notice the differences that take place in the previously locked area and in the rest of your body. ✎

FIBROMYALGIA

Fibromyalgia is a condition that affects millions of Americans, the majority of whom are women. These individuals suffer from an array of symptoms, primarily persistent muscular pain. Many of these people also suffer from chronic fatigue, irritable bowel syndrome, and spastic colon. Still other individuals may be afflicted with migraines, severe premenstrual syndrome, and even heart arrhythmias.

At one time, the medical model attributed fibromyalgia to "psychosomatic" origins—in other words, that it was "all in your head." These sorts of labels were counterproductive and did little more than "blame the victim." They dismissed patients, who had very real symptoms, as hypochondriacs and malingerers, implying that they were basically imagining their complaints.

Now that the tide is finally turning, many researchers are looking for viral, biochemical, and genetic causation to fibromyalgia. Yet, as is often the case when the pendulum swings, the truth has been passed over in the race for the new breakthrough. While we can't rule out molecular and genetic influences, the current opposing psychosomatic-versus-biological explanations have largely missed the mark and are of limited value in suggesting effective treatment.

From the perspective of this program, one of the most important underlying factors in fibromyalgia is the stuck fight/flight/freeze (i.e. trauma) reaction. Simply put, the unreleased muscle tensing leads to pain, which leads, in turn, to fear and more bracing, and more pain, and so on. When enough of this pain affects enough of the body, people are diagnosed (somewhat arbitrarily) with "fibromyalgia."

Neglect and abuse are powerful factors in predisposing the development of fibromyalgia. Another important component of fibromyalgia is repressed anger. In general, traumatized individuals are afraid to feel their anger and own their healthy aggression.

In seeking resolution to the pain, you must proceed ever-so-slowly and carefully because of the severity of symptoms, particularly if they involve the gastrointestinal system, migraines, or severe PMS. At the same time it is essential that you consult an internist, as some of these symptoms might conceivably be due to an organic cause. Keep in mind that as you begin to release some of this locked-in energy, there may be a temporary exacerbation of your symptoms. Less is more, so proceed at your own self-compassionate pace. At any time, if you feel that working with your symptoms may be too much, please seek a therapist, particularly one trained in Somatic Experiencing or another modality that works effectively in a very gentle way. Trust your instincts and intuition to find the right therapist for *you;* no matter how many diplomas they may have hanging on their wall, rely on your *feelings* about who is right for you.

Helen: A Forgotten Moment

Helen had begun to show the early signs of fibromyalgia. While this was causing her concern, this was not the reason she sought consultation.

She came to the office because of emotions that she could not "understand." Her friends had become concerned that she was increasingly submissive and unpredictably explosive. At the point when her behavior threatened her relations with friends and colleagues, she too became concerned. Helen did not make the connection between her physical and behavioral changes and an event that had transpired three years earlier, which, as far as she was concerned, was irrelevant.

I asked Helen to recall a recent encounter with a colleague that illustrated her sudden shift in behavior. We both noted Helen's bodily reactions as she recounted the event. I noticed that her shoulders were high and "hunched over" and brought that to Helen's attention. She reported that her shoulder and neck were getting tight and painful. "It's like the pain I feel when I am under stress." Helen then said that she felt that she had done something wrong. I asked if this was a feeling or a thought. After a moment Helen replied: "I think it's a thought." We both giggled. Very often we are not aware that we are having a thought. Frequently we confuse our thoughts with reality, rather than realizing they're just thoughts. I then asked her to bring her attention to her body. She reported a sinking sensation in her belly. "It makes me hate myself." Helen was taken aback by this sudden outburst of self-loathing.

Rather than analyzing *why* she felt that way, I guided her back to the sensations in her body. After a pause, Helen reported that her "heart and mind were racing a million miles an hour." She then became disturbed by what she described as a "sweaty, smelly, hot sensation" on her back, which left her feeling nauseated. The pain in her neck and shoulders intensified to a 7.5 on a pain scale of 10. The pain, she said, "is driving me crazy." Helen now seemed more agitated—her face turned pale and she felt an urge to get up and leave the room. After reassurance, Helen continued tracking her discomfort. The pain intensified again, and then gradually diminished. Following this ebb and flow, Helen became aware of another sensation—a more specific tension in the back of her right arm and shoulder.

When she focused her attention on this sensation, she started to feel an urge to thrust her elbow backward. I offered a hand as a support and as a resistance so that Helen could safely feel the power in her arm as she gently pushed it slowly backward. After pushing for several seconds, her body began to shake and tremble. Her legs also began to move slowly up and down as if they were on a sewing machine treadle, or as though she were running.

As Helen's arm continued to slowly press backwards, the shaking decreased and she felt as though her legs were getting stronger. "They feel like they want to move," she said. Helen then reported noticing a strong urge propelling her forward. Suddenly, a picture flashed before her: a street lamp and the image of a couple who had helped her. "I got away . . . I got away . . . " she cried softly. It was then she remembered molding into the man's torso as he held a knife to her throat. She went on, "I did that to make him think I was his . . . then my body knew what to do and it did it . . . that's what let me escape."

The story that her body had been telling then emerged in words: three years earlier, Helen had been the victim of an attempted rape. While she was walking home after visiting a friend in an unfamiliar neighborhood, a stranger had pulled her into an alley and threatened to kill her if she didn't cooperate. Somehow, she was able to break free and run to a lighted street corner where two passersby yelled for the police. Helen was politely interviewed by the police and then taken home by her friend. Surprisingly, she could not remember how she had escaped, but was tearfully grateful to have been left unharmed. Afterward, her life appeared to return to normal, but when she felt stressed or in conflict, her body was still responding as it had when the knife was held to her throat. Her body was bearing the burden in the form of chronic pain.

Helen found herself helpless and passive or easily enraged under everyday stress, not "realizing" that this was a replay of the brief pretense at submissiveness that had probably saved her life. Her "submission" successfully fooled the assailant, allowing a momentary opportunity for the instinctual energy of a wild animal to take over, propelling her arms and legs in a successful escape. However, it had all happened so fast that she had not had the chance to integrate the experience. At a primitive body level, she still didn't "know" that she had escaped, and remained identified with the submissiveness rather than with her complete two-phase strategy that had in fact saved her life. Somatically and emotionally, it was as if part of her was still in the assailant's clutches.

After processing and completing the rape-related actions, Helen now reported having an overall sense of "capability" and empowerment. In place of the previous submissive self-hatred, she was "back to even more of her (old) self." This new self came from being able to *physically feel* the motor response of elbowing her assailant, and then *sense* the immense power in her legs, which had carried her to safety. Helen realized that the painful tension in her neck, shoulders, and legs was the energy needed to protect herself, energy that got stuck. In her words, "It released like waves of warm tingly vibration." She had made a major step in freeing herself from the prison of chronic pain. In the following weeks her symptoms lessened, and though she had some flare-ups, her symptoms gradually disappeared. Helen's fibromyalgia was mild, and her early childhood history of trauma was relatively minor; it should be noted that in most cases of fibromyalgia changes occur more slowly over time.

How many of our habitual behaviors and feelings are outside of our conscious awareness or are long *accepted* as part of ourselves, of who we are, when in fact they are not? Often, these behaviors are reactions to events long forgotten or rationalized by our minds, but remembered accurately by our bodies. Sigmund Freud once said: "The mind has forgotten but the body has not, thankfully." We can thank Freud for correctly surmising that both the imprints of horrible experiences as well as their antidotes—in the form of resiliency and the capacity for forming new experiences that lead to transformation—exist within our living, feeling, knowing bodies.

Possibilities for Working with Anger and Other Emotions that Underlie Chronic Pain and Fibromyalgia

Results with Helen were achieved when she could *safely* feel and release her anger and re-own her sense of self-protection. Here are some ways you can try this approach for yourself.

Sit comfortably and slowly push your legs into the ground. To do so, you might want to place both feet on the floor, making sure that the rest of your body is supported—whether you are lying or sitting.

As you breathe in, feel your energy rise through your core, and as you breathe out, press down gently through your feet (see the grounding exercise on page 33 or audio track 4). Experiment for a few breath cycles; if this is not helping you feel more grounded, reverse the directions (pressing down through your feet and legs as you breathe in and letting go as you breathe out). Notice what you begin to feel.

Sense any anger you might be aware of related to fibromyalgia or another pain condition. Imagine the movements your body might want to make to express this frustration, anger, or irritability. For example, you might perceive pushing or chopping motions, or sense an impulse to move your arm to strike out.

Allow this movement to occur very, very slowly so that you can integrate all the subtleties that take place. As examples, allow your hands to push forward very slowly, feeling each movement; or allow your hands to make slow motions, gentle karate chops into a pillow.

You can also add resistance by placing a soft, thick
pillow against the wall (or better still, asking a friend
to hold the pillow) as you gradually push into it.

It is important to move *gradually* to complete the action of healthy
aggression, and thereby release the stuck survival energy that is locked
in your muscles and nervous system. The key is to *feel* yourself completing the full range of the movement and *directing* the movement. It
isn't enough to mindlessly or mechanically karate chop a pillow. You
must *feel* what it is like to prepare for the strike, align your spine with
the strike, and come down with the intention of cutting through that
obstacle—and then *feel* your hand successfully shear through the pillow.

Give yourself time to stop and integrate what you have experienced.
How does your body feel different? When you think about the stimu-
lus for your anger, how is your reaction different now? You may want
to record what you are noticing in your pain journal so that you can
come back to this when you feel anger activation again. ✐

MIGRAINE HEADACHES

Migraine headaches arise from a fundamental dysregulation of the autonomic nervous system. What's known about migraines is that they seem
to be caused first by a constricting of the blood vessels in the head, followed by a precipitous dilation, or expansion, of these blood vessels. It is
this abrupt stretching that causes the pain.

To reduce the severity of migraines, it's important to focus on what
happens *before* the migraine, especially the preliminary signals that
occur just before you recognize its onset. This is sometimes called the
prodromal stage of migraine. Often, people with migraines will identify flickering lights, an aura, a certain feeling or sensation, a taste or
even a smell prior to the onset of the full migraine. When they learn
how to become aware of what happens just before the first symptom
appears, they generally find that the attack doesn't occur or at least

is diminished We have found that the majority of individuals who practice mindful awareness and tracking of sensations have gotten significant relief with the frequency and severity of their migraine symptoms. This type of work must be conducted at a careful pace, because symptoms like migraines have a great deal of locked-in energy that requires gradual release.

Donna: Out of the Frying Pan *and* the Fire

Donna had struggled with migraines off and on during the last ten years. Her only child, Sam, had recently graduated from college and was out on his own. She and her husband were now empty nesters who had frequent surges of tension as old conflicts resurfaced in more intense forms without the buffering that their son Sam had provided.

In the last two years, Donna's migraines had worsened as she moved into perimenopause. She had tried several medications without significant results, and acupuncture brought only temporary relief. At the time she sought treatment, she was missing an average of half a day a week at work because of the unmanageable pain. She was becoming concerned about losing her job, a worry that increased her complaints of anxiety as well as the frequency of migraines.

Donna's history revealed several traumatic events related to men, beginning with her father, who had had numerous affairs and a gambling addiction. This situation had thrown the family into bankruptcy. She also reported an attempted date rape in high school by her boyfriend of two years, and feelings of betrayal because of her husband's flirtations early in their marriage. A trial of couple counseling at that time had had little long-term benefit.

Although Donna was motivated and quite eager to relieve her headaches, it was very difficult for her to connect with her body sensations. In fact, her body was the enemy, the source of pain that was also holding on to excess weight (related to medications and hormonal fluctuations). "I don't want to get to know my body," she said. "I understand from what you've told me that I cannot recover from migraines without being able to feel what's happening so I can prevent the full attacks, but all I feel is disgust." After learning about mindfulness, however, Donna was more hopeful. "I've heard about this approach and I'd like to try it."

Her first attempts at practicing mindfulness were often interrupted by self-judgment and obsessive negative thinking. She participated in several mindfulness sessions, using tools similar to the exercise that follows. Eventually, Donna was able to lower her pain a point or two when she chose to lie down and practice steady, balanced breathing. This success helped her to track sensations that seemed to underlie the pain. She was ultimately able to utilize her obsessive-thinking style as a skill to help her name and write down each sensation that occurred. This self-designed practice allowed her to connect enough with her body to move through each migraine episode—each time with a little more ease.

Gradually, she was able to identify the earliest signs of a migraine, which for her were throbbing sensations in her temples followed by feelings of pressure in the front of her head. She used these warning signals as opportunities to lower her stress at work or at home, including requesting that her husband prepare meals so she could rest.

Donna's approach suggests a strategy you might try. Like Donna, when you notice sensations that herald the beginning of a pain episode, you can remind yourself that these are frequently signs that a migraine or other pain symptom might be approaching. At that point, if at home, you can train yourself to ask family members to prepare meals or complete other chores, so you can lie down for an hour or so to use the tools you know to lessen the pain. If the symptoms occur at work, you can practice shifting to less demanding tasks or ask a team member for help.

Gradually, using these strategies, Donna's headaches diminished in intensity and frequency. "I still have migraines," she reported at our last session, "but I know I can rest and I know that I can bring the pain down. What I have now that I did not have before is peace of mind."

EXERCISE: Mindfulness-Based Pain-Relief Practice
🔊 Track 15

Mindfulness-based practice can be useful with any kind of pain. If you'd like to explore this, find a comfortable position where your body feels supported and where you are relatively free from distraction.

Begin by using one of the tools you have learned thus far from the Freedom from Pain program that helps you connect safely and comfortably with your body. For example, go back to the Just One Breath exercise on page 33 (audio track 5) and/or work with the Securing a Resting Place in Your Body exercise on page 31 (audio track 3).

Then, when you're ready to begin exploring this exercise, imagine that you can step into a new moment with beginner's mind as if for the very first time. Begin to notice what you find in this new moment.

Take an inventory of your thoughts, feelings, sensations, inner images, movements in your body, posture, and gestures. Describe them out loud. For example: "Now I feel that pressure in my temples and notice that my vision is beginning to change like it does before a migraine." Or with another type of pain: "Right now, I can feel a burning in my left leg, a cramping in my stomach, and I have the thought that I'm discouraged. I don't think I can get past this pain."

When you reach a natural pause in the flow of your awareness, take a deep breath in and hold it; then allow yourself to accept, with kindness and compassion, that you feel a pressure in your temples and a blurring and narrowing of your vision (or burning in your left leg, a cramping in your stomach, or the thought that you're discouraged because you don't think you can make it through this). Accept the thought, and accept the pain. Hold all of the awarenesses that you have named along with your breath . . . and when you're ready . . . let them all go as you breathe out.

Then with the next breath in, step into the next new moment as if for the very first time. Explore this new moment and name for yourself what you're aware of at that point; for example: "I'm still feeling the pressure in my temples and the changes in my vision, except the pressure is lighter and there is now a pulsing in the back of my head." Another possibility might be, "I'm still feeling the burning in my left leg, only it's moved down into my lower leg," and so on.

When you sense a pause or completion, take a deep breath in and hold it while you accept with kindness and gentleness toward yourself whatever you're experiencing. Vocalize what you are sensing and feeling. For example, maybe the pressure has lightened and the pulsing is slowing. Or the burning in your left leg has moved lower, you still have the stomach cramping, and you're wondering, "Can I really make it through all of this? Will I have a normal life again?" Hold your breath along with all of these thoughts and feelings and when you're ready, let it all go along with your breath as you exhale.

Continue this process of accepting what you are experiencing, naming what you are aware of, then holding your breath and releasing all of your experience through your out-breath; then return to your body with the next new inhalation as if it were the very first time.

You can continue to explore mindfully additional, new moments in this way until you reach a sense of completion or readiness to stop the exercise. Generally, less is more—so no need to push yourself. Also, check in and review your progress as you continue this exercise over time. What has happened during the time you've been practicing this mindfulness exercise regularly? What is different about your sense of pain? Do you experience more energy, or feel an enhanced sense of aliveness? Are you noticing more fluid shifts between constriction and expansion in your body? We encourage you to record your experiences with this exercise in your pain journal. ✐

There are many types of mindfulness exercises that can help you strengthen your awareness of sensation in your body. Coupling non-judgmental thoughts with sensate awareness (body awareness), and using your breath to open pathways in your body, can help you shift your discomfort into a dynamic flow of self-discovery.

INTERSTITIAL CYSTITIS

Interstitial cystitis, sometimes called *bladder pain syndrome,* is a disorder characterized by pain associated with urination or with increased urinary frequency (often as frequently as every ten minutes). There is also urgency and/or pressure in the bladder and even in much of the pelvis. It is more common in women than men. With men, mild cases are often associated with pain or difficulty when urinating in a public bathroom. For both men and women, it is exacerbated by stress.[1] A Harvard University study concluded that "the impact of interstitial cystitis on quality of life is severe and debilitating."[2] The condition is now officially recognized as a disability.

The cause of this disorder seems to be complex and is largely unknown. However, we believe it is due to a sympathetic nervous (fight/flight) system constriction of the smooth muscle in the bladder and urinary tract. Exposure to childhood trauma is associated with a six-fold increased risk of developing the disorder—about the same correlation as with fibromyalgia, chronic fatigue, and irritable bowel syndrome. As many as 70 percent of these individuals have suffered physical and/or emotional abuse as compared to 15 percent of healthy individuals.[3] And this is not even taking into account other traumas such as medical traumas and accidents. There are strong indications that both irritable bladder and fibromyalgia are trauma related.

The various breathing and pendulation exercises you have practiced for other pain syndromes are applicable to this disorder as well. In addition, we suggest you try sitting on a gymnastic ball with your feet shoulder-width apart, contacting the floor to maintain an easy balance. Then become aware of how the ball contacts and supports the floor of your pelvis as you breathe in. With your out-breath, just allow the floor of your pelvis to sink into the ball. This particular exercise is often quite useful in working with PMS and other types of pelvic pain.

CHRONIC REGIONAL PAIN SYNDROME

One of the most challenging pain conditions is reflex sympathetic dystrophy (RSD), which is now, generally, called chronic regional pain syndrome (CRPS). It is another pain condition related to regulatory problems in the autonomic nervous system. Sometimes the pain is in one part of the body and will appear to generate a freezing cold sensation, while another part of the body will feel burning hot. These temperatures can actually be felt on the outside of the body as well as on the inside. This kind of pain is called "exquisite pain." The word "exquisite" is used here in a negative sense, as in "exquisitely painful."

One approach that has been very successful with CRPS/RSD is the use of very light touch across the limb, joint, or area involved. Some Somatic Experiencing therapists have developed this method. In this case, touch is used to help amplify a person's ability to get under the pain and experience their underlying non-pain sensations, while also providing support to the individual to keep exploring.

An example of this approach was used with Michael, a ninety-two-year old man diagnosed with neuropathy, which is often one of the symptoms of CRPS. He had classic symptoms in his extremities—burning sensations in his arms, hands, legs, and feet. He was guided to do some simple tracking of sensations, and two incidents came up which greatly surprised him. Michael had been a marine under fire during World War II and, many years later, also survived a fatality-causing tornado that threatened his home. He had never talked to anyone about these experiences. He had difficulties feeling into the pain, typically reporting "feeling nothing" or "feeling the same." Eventually, he noticed that when he achieved awareness of the sensations related to these two traumatic events, and amplified them slowly through touching these areas gently with his hands, his pain level went from 8 to a pain level of between 2 and 3.

The typical medical thinking is that neuropathy and other types of CRPS cannot be reversed. Many medical practitioners tend to be very frustrated about CRPS, sometimes even venting anger with comments like, "Wait a minute, what's going on here? Your pain was in your left knee last week, now you say it's in your right hip?!" The shifting from place to place in the body, known as migrating pain, may be an expression of involuntary dysregulation in the autonomic nervous system. Our position is that even if this kind of pain is caused by some structural change in the tissues, when the patient can achieve better self-regulation, pain levels can dramatically change.

It's really important to appreciate that CRPS is not all in your head. Knowledge can be empowering, especially if you understand that migrating pain has a cause, and that the cause is not that something is wrong with you, but occurs because of the pervasive dysregulation. There are special skills that you need to learn in order to work with these elusive pain sensations to achieve regulation and relief.

Possibilities for Working with CRPS

One effective way of working with CRPS or other types of migrating pain is to learn to connect the different sensations and regions of the body that are linked with pain. The following is an exercise that can be used whether you have CRPS or other types of pain that affect different parts of your body.

Take a few moments now to explore various areas of discomfort. If helpful, use your hands to gently touch those areas of your body as Michael was taught to do. Place your hand gently on one area at a time and imagine that you can breathe into it very gently. Notice what shifts with the sensations.

Then practice a special kind of pendulation (see page 69) by connecting these pain areas together. For example, if you are experiencing pain in your foot and also along the sciatic nerve and in your lower back, take time to breathe into one area and then, one by one, into the others. Now use your attention and focus to move from one of these locations to another. For example, you could first bridge from your foot to the sciatic area, noticing the effects that occur, then shift back and forth several times, noting what becomes different. Next, you could bridge from your sciatic area to your lower back, going back and forth between each of these two locations several times.

Finally, use your breath to help this along. Breathe in when you connect with one location, then breathe out when you connect with the second (or the reverse: breathe in when you connect with the second and out when linking to the first area). What do you notice after shifting in this way?

If needed, you can add an area of relative comfort or neutrality as one of your bridging destinations. What difference does this resource make? You may want to take a little time to write about your experiences of this mini-exercise in your pain journal.

CHRONIC DEPRESSION

Chronic depression is emotional pain often related to separation, loss, abandonment, and insecure attachment relationships. Depression can also be a byproduct of chronic pain because we can become worn down by intense and unrelenting discomfort. Since depression so often accompanies many pain conditions, antidepressants are often included in pain treatment protocols.

The biggest challenge involved in resolving depression is to thaw the freeze or immobility response on a daily basis by mobilizing toward action within your body and in your greater life. Taking a fifteen to twenty minute walk a couple of times a day can begin to make a difference. It's helpful to understand that depression, especially when viewed from its close relationship to the freeze response, is a way of shutting down as a "last-ditch" form of protection. Although there is no specific way of determining whether a given case of depression is linked to unresolved immobility, some of the signs of this connection are a lower blood pressure and slower heart rate and respiration under stress. Dizziness and light-headedness can also be symptoms.

When SSRIs (selective serotonin reuptake inhibitors) such as Prozac came into mainstream use, experts suggested that depression must be a disorder of insufficient serotonin. Although there's some truth to this premise, what's interesting is that a brisk walk around the block can elevate serotonin levels as effectively as medication. There is no cost involved in walking—nor are there any bothersome side effects.

You might begin by making choices that allow you to be more active in your body, such as gentle stretching, practicing simple yoga poses, or taking a short walk when you would rather collapse and lie in bed. Even more effective is to engage in action that involves the company of another person, such as playing with a child, going to a "safe" non-triggering movie, or dancing to your preferred type of music. In this case, activity is especially important at times when you least feel like being active.

Taking action to raise serotonin levels is only part of the solution, however. People who use exercise (or anti-depressants) to help regulate their neurotransmitters may become less depressed, but sometimes will experience more anxiety. The question then becomes how to deal effectively with the anxiety that often surfaces so as not to flip back into the depression.

Possibilities for Working with Depression and Emerging Anxiety

It is important to develop simple, effective ways of self-soothing that allow you to access a sense of safety, strength, and support through your body experience, and which support movement into safe action. For example, if you have a friend or partner who is willing to help you, ask that person to stand facing you partly, with one leg in front of the other for support, and offer you one or both hands for you to push against with your hand (or

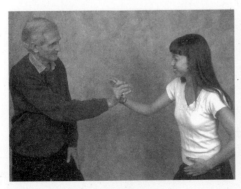

Figure A

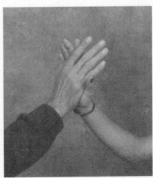

Figure B

hands). If it feels safe to do so, you can name what you are pushing against that triggers a depressive reaction in you (for example, pain, discouragement, a critical boss, or a mysterious new pain symptom).[4]

Naturally, if your pain increases, stop and rest. Debrief afterward by communicating what you experienced. You might want to write about this practice session in your pain journal: specifically, what did you learn about how to work with your depression?

Although breathing techniques can be very helpful with depression, deep breathing techniques sometimes cause an increase in anxiety, and can even incite a greater collapse into depression or helplessness. So understand that if this happens, just rest and then try it again, if you like. Very often, just a few moments of rest is all that it takes for your nervous system to come one more step out of the depression. In addition to circle breathing (see the exercise on page 24), you can also learn to create a body safe place by first identifying a place in your body that is a little more comfortable than any other. Once you find this, breathe gently and normally into that area of the body to better connect with a sense of safety or strength or comfort. With practice over time, your body safe place can become a touchstone for connection that is reliably positive.

Since depression is linked with the freeze response, as the response begins to "thaw," different layers of distress, including hyperarousal, rage, grief, or fear may surface. In these cases, it is often helpful to use the breath to regulate the distress by voicing a sound such as "voo" during a slow exhalation. This tends to help titrate or naturally dilute the surfacing emotions that often can feel overwhelming and uncontrollable. (See Voo Breathing exercise on page 34.)

To help further with a hyperactivated or anxious state that can emerge when the freeze of the depression begins to shift, you can use the same pushing practice with a partner described earlier to gently release the anxiety.

Rage and aggression are also commonly connected with depression. Studies and clinical observation have indicated that some types of depression are caused by rage turned inward against the self. It's very important to know how to work with rage in a contained way. Imagery can be very helpful in beginning to process rage in a safe way. Following is a useful application of imagery. Even though this is a fantasy, it can be unsettling at first. If it seems too much for you, just skip over it for now.

Ask yourself the question, "If my rage could be expressed right now, what might that look like? What color might it be? What would it want to do? Who (or what) would be the target of my anger?"

Sometimes, just by looking from a distance at one aspect of your anger or aggression, you can envision or fantasize expressing it. Would you like to pound the source of your anger to a pulp? Would you like to cut it up with a knife, or stomp on it until nothing is left, until it is completely destroyed? As you connect with any of these images, what do you notice in your body right now?

Working with aggression and impulses with the goal of complete destruction at least allows the acceptance of these taboo emotions. Then you can begin to understand that rage is indeed linked to the impulse to destroy, but is also a *feeling* and an *image* of destroying. This is different than actually hurting someone else or hurting yourself. So while the imagery can be a bit scary at first, with a little creative practice, it can become exhilarating.

In addition to channeling aggression and dealing with anger (in resolving depression), the most important interventions are related to helping you develop the skills to socialize and accept social support. This allows your ventral vagal,[5] or social engagement system, to re-engage and provides additional resources to counter the depressive, isolating tendencies that can take you back into the state of freeze and collapse. The right kind of support group can be invaluable in reinforcing and strengthening social skills. I once led a pain group, and by the end of the night, we were all laughing uncontrollably at each other's gallows humor. Such laughter, by the way, is a great way to release endorphins, the body's built-in pain control agents.

If you are frozen in chronic depression, it is necessary to take very small steps toward recovery. Maybe you can begin by discovering what gives you even a tiny bit of pleasure, or what is at least reliably neutral. If you cannot find this small island of "OK-ness," a professional might help you to learn to take small actions to generate new experience. Also medications can sometimes give people enough of a lift to mobilize them to use the Freedom from Pain tools more effectively.

Are you willing just one time when you get up in the morning to put on some gentle music to accompany some slow easy movements and stretching instead of going back to bed, just to find out what that feels like? We can't predict how that will feel to you, but do you have anything to lose? We can predict how constricted life will remain if you continue to follow your usual patterns.

It's also important to remember that there may be a great deal of shame embedded in depression. Shame is often coupled with helplessness and collapse. You may feel shame in asking for or receiving the level of help and support you really need and in allowing others to see your imperfections and helplessness. Feeling shame can send you deeper into a state of withdrawal and collapse. Learning to identify, feel, and regulate the sensations related to shame, however, can help decrease your pain and depression.

Working Mindfully with Chronic Depression

One of the most effective types of intervention with chronic depression, as with chronic pain, is mindfulness. An example is learning to develop what psychologist and lay Buddhist priest Tara Brach calls "radical self-acceptance."[6] This is a truly radical practice because at the moment that you are least able to give yourself acceptance, you are called on to give complete and authentic acceptance to yourself, which can result in a conflict-free moment of acceptance and love for yourself.

Here's a three-step method that can help you develop radical self-acceptance. First, you must be willing to pause and notice that you are not accepting yourself . . . and *to accept your lack of acceptance* for the time being. There are a number of ways to notice this: there's the voice you hear in your mind telling you that you're no good, or you may find yourself disconnecting or dissociating from body experience when you don't want to accept or feel it. Another way might be to notice the unwanted shame triggered by devaluing social interactions that make you think that you are worthless or unlovable, thus compounding the lack of self-acceptance you feel. This first step, called the "sacred pause," is often the most challenging. You must be willing to stop, as Brach suggests, and simply notice your lack of acceptance.

Step two is to make an inner commitment to turn your mind toward some form of acceptance, whatever is possible at a given moment. For example, you can shift from "I am worthless" to "I feel worthwhile when I am at work, or when I am with my children."

And step three is to continue to repeat the first two steps as long as it's helpful. Understandably, like life itself, this is an endless practice. You might want to work with this as a mini-practice exercise and note your results in your pain journal. The following exercise may also provide additional practice for you. ✒

EXERCISE: Finding the Energy to Resolve Depression

One practical example of how to turn your mind toward self-acceptance is derived from what is called Energy Psychology. This technique is used to clear *reversals*, which in energy terms are disturbances that usually come from an inner conflict where the person is both moving toward a positive change and moving away from this change at the same time.

To clear an energy reversal, we use positive self-affirmations while stimulating specific energy points along one of the meridians or energy pathways in your body. To practice this, find your so-called neurolymphatic points by feeling your collarbone at your neckline, then coming toward the midline of your body, from that point moving one inch down toward your feet on the left side (or both sides), and then over four to six inches toward your shoulder. If you encounter the fold of the shoulder, you've gone too far. If you rub in the correct area, you'll usually feel tenderness.[7] (If these directions sound confusing, please see diagrams referenced in the endnote to clarify this practice.)

The approach is to rub these points on either side of the chest (but especially on the left side) because this is believed to help release toxins and stress. As you rub those points on your chest, you say a simple affirmation such as, "I deeply and completely love and accept myself, even with all my problems and limitations." This clearing technique requires you to say this or another similar phrase three times.

The affirmation works because it expresses your positive intentions toward yourself even if you are not able to actualize them or believe them yet. You can also add other specific affirmations like, "I deeply and completely love and accept myself even though I don't *think* I'll ever be free of depression" or "I deeply and completely love and accept myself even though I hate the way I am right now," or whatever is true at the moment. It's important to word the main affirmation so that you can really resonate with it; for example, "I *want* to deeply and completely love and accept myself" or "I *wish I could* deeply and completely love and accept myself."

The Science of Affirmations

We can understand why affirmations work by examining research conducted in neuroplasticity, which has demonstrated that our physical reality is formed from past experience.

In other words, whatever symptoms or problems we have, including pain, as well as whatever strengths we have, are much more based on experience than we ever thought was true. Most of us subscribe to the theory that DNA genetically determines who and how we are in the world. Neuroplasticity research has turned this theory on its head and gives us an entirely new way to look at the impact of our thoughts and beliefs.

We know that thoughts literally change brain chemistry. Research indicates that the chemical composition of the body can change in relation to a specific thought within twenty seconds.[8] This shift can be measured in a number of surprising ways. One way is to measure the acid or alkaline effect the thought has on the body.

If we're really focused on a negative thought or limiting belief, our nervous system will send messages almost immediately to our muscles, which will then constrict. Negative thoughts affect our thinking mind as well so that we can't think well and can also increase anxiety. In addition to external threats that can activate the freeze of depression, we also need to be aware of internal threats, such as negative thoughts or negative beliefs coming from inside us.

Cells in the brain that fire together get wired together. If we have thought or experiential connections that aren't used very much, those will be eliminated. Those brain cells that are wired together create a neuronal network; in the case of affirmations, a positive "higher self" network is generated that can automatically be set off when we encounter a negative trigger in everyday life. So affirmations can bring important changes in self-acceptance if you use them only a few times. If you use them regularly, you'll get even more results because they create a special wiring and firing pattern that results in a new neuronal network.[9]

Marti: A Mindful Path to the Pain-Free Self

Marti has struggled with depression for as long as she can remember. Her mother was hospitalized with severe postpartum depression just after Marti's birth and her grandmother took care of her during that time. Marti's sense was that the roots of her own depression were in the loss of her nurturing grandmother and the intrusion of her mother's anxiety when she returned to the home several months later. Marti had fragmentary images of both her mother and her father physically abusing her throughout her childhood.

As an adult, Marti became a competent attorney in human rights, yet in her early forties, she developed fibromyalgia, chronic fatigue, migraine headaches, and severe depression. Although antidepressant medication helped her somewhat, Marti continued to struggle with this quartet of syndromes and ultimately went on disability because she could no longer work.

As we explored the connections between these health problems, we decided to use affirmations to begin to shift these patterns in an attempt to boost her energy system. The affirmations that seemed to work best for her included: "I deeply and completely love and accept myself even though I'm depressed and have pain most of the time"; "I deeply and completely love myself even though most of my life I have believed I'm unlovable . . . I forgive myself for this conclusion"; "I deeply and completely appreciate myself even though my family has never known how to appreciate me."

Marti found that she could remember to say the affirmations while rubbing the neurolymphatic point on her left chest whenever she felt her pain and depression increase. Although the positive results were subtle and slow, over time she felt more stable and was able to decrease the dosage on both her antidepressant and pain medications. She began exercising and then used the affirmations to manage the pain flare-ups that sometimes resulted. Marti's evaluation was that "many tools helped me to reclaim my health, but the affirmations were easy to remember to use and brought instant relief. I could use them in just about any situation and the results were almost always positive."

Practicing Affirmations

If you'd like to practice using affirmations to help you manage your depression and pain, take a few minutes and try out a few basic ones. It's good to start with the basic phrase, "I deeply and completely love, accept, and appreciate myself even though . . . (add your own words here)." Leading with a positive affirmation allows you to hold your depression and pain in a more balanced and positive way.

Practice using your affirmations for several days when you are aware of an increase in pain or depression. Make sure the words you choose fully resonate with your body. What changes do you notice? Note your results in your pain journal.

Don't be discouraged when you don't get immediate results from your affirmation. Once I felt completely overwhelmed by the vast amount of work I had to complete, while at the same time I had a wrist injury that was aggravated by typing. When I thought about trying an affirmation, I heard the words in my mind, "That won't do any good, you just have to do it." Then the following affirmation spontaneously arose in my mind: "I can ask for help, I don't have to do it alone." I chuckled and then called a friend and asked if he would be willing to type as I dictated. The specific affirmations that you will find for yourself are limited only by your imagination, creativity, and willingness to seek ways to promote your healing process.

CHAPTER SIX

Preventing and Resolving the Pain of Medical Trauma

MANY PEOPLE IN PAIN struggle with the dilemma that the very medical procedures and practices designed to help them recover often create additional pain and are thus potentially traumatizing. This happens because the fear and pain that can occur before, during, and after surgery (and other invasive medical procedures) are frequently not adequately managed.

The reality is that much of what happens for the sake of diagnosing and treating your pain is invasive—the body unconsciously perceives it as an attack. Even while under anesthesia, your peripheral nerves are still active, as is your autonomic nervous system (which keeps your heart beating, your lungs breathing, and so forth). More importantly, the threat detectors in your nervous system are still at work. Sensors in your skin, muscles, and viscera are sending threat messages to the so-called "primitive" brain stem.

If you were mugged by a thug with a knife, or attacked in a back alley with a syringe full of poison, you would consider this a criminal assault.

However, a doctor may plunge a needle into tissue around a joint to remove painful, excess fluid, saw through the bones of your leg to replace a crumbling hip, or even flood much of your body with poison to kill cancerous cells. The brain stem cannot discern the intentions behind a sensation of pain or cutting, only that it exists. So even if the sensations associated with a surgery are intended to heal, the body may perceive little difference between them and the sensations of being attacked and torn apart.

Within the framework of medicine, most of us willingly schedule and expend large amounts of money for these kinds of intrusive procedures because we trust the skill of well-trained professionals and assume that the alternatives—a life of pain, illness, incapacity, or even death—are far worse. Yet we often don't respect the severity of the consequences that result from these invasions.

There's no doubt that many pain-reducing procedures, including surgery, are successful and improve quality of life for many people. Problems ensue, however, when we are not properly prepared for the possibilities of severe pain related to the medical procedure itself or the emotional suffering that results when our expectations for improvement in our condition are not immediately met.

In this chapter, we want to help prepare you for these kinds of situations, and for the process of working with medical professionals in order to prevent and resolve the traumatic effects of invasive treatments that have the potential to increase or sustain your pain. Once again, our message is that your success is largely up to *you*—your positive attitude, your motivation and willingness to prepare as thoroughly as you would for other challenges in life, and your ability to communicate effectively with your treatment team.

EXAMINE AND USE YOUR RESOURCES AND STRENGTHS

We'd like to start with the suggestion that you take time to inventory the *resources* you bring to any medical intervention that has the potential to increase or decrease your pain. In other words, rather than beginning with the fears or problems you anticipate, we encourage you to begin with your strengths and your trust in the medical team that is serving you. These kinds of resources can serve as points of strengths and support to buffer against possible trouble. Especially when you are going into an unfamiliar situation that you've never encountered, it's best to draw on what has already worked well for you in dealing with the usual challenges of daily life or even prior medical situations. It's important to honor whatever approach helps you to feel comfortable and safe.

For example, some people excel in athletics and have learned to rely on the strength and stamina of their "can-do" bodies. This is a benefit, because their bodies are typically stronger and tend to bounce back more quickly from serious procedures like surgeries. Others are more inclined toward meditative and creative capacities. For them, playing music, writing, painting, or inward focusing helps to create a sense of calm support and centered relaxation. Still others tend to be more intellectual, preferring to research things exhaustively, preparing for their procedures like they would a test. And then there are other folks who find they benefit most from getting immersed in diversions, like movies or computer games.

Miriam, for example, was a graphic design artist, and her ability to visualize helped facilitate her recovery from hand surgery. Each time she thought about the procedure, she imagined the steady hands of her surgeon as he worked with confidence in his skills and the understanding of how important it was for her to recover full function of her hands. Miriam envisioned her recovery as a gradual emergence from the anesthetic and the normal soreness of minor surgery. She also created a series of mental graphics to illustrate her progression from soreness, stiffness, and pale skin, indicating the freeze response, to pink, healthy tissues and ongoing return of flexibility.

Work from your strengths, using whatever works best for you, to help ease the fearful, angry, as well as panicky reactions that might arise. If you feel comforted by extensive research and study of the procedure you have chosen, honor that. On the other hand, if you tend to feel overwhelmed by reading the reactions of others and the opinions of different professionals on the Internet or other formats, honor your need to restrict the kind of input that may increase your worry.

During the time of gathering and organizing information, it is also important to balance whatever anxiety and fears emerge with positive facts like the success rates of the surgery, the number of procedures the doctor has performed successfully, and reminders of the ways you've responded in other situations where you've needed to heal.

An important type of resource is made available by reviewing past positive medical experiences. How well and how quickly did you recover? How did you get through any complications? What do you think helped you recover? How could you use those same strategies now? Reminders of the ways you've responded in other situations where you've needed to heal will ensure a smoother recovery. You might want to explore these questions in your pain journal so you can refer back to them. ✐

BUILD SAFETY BY GETTING
THE RIGHT KIND OF INFORMATION

In order to make a good informed decision about the surgery or other procedure, it is important to gather the type of information that can increase your confidence. It's usually best to start with the professional who is performing the treatment. Make sure that you have the opportunity to meet *in person* with the actual surgeon or individual who will be implementing the intervention. Take stock of whether your concerns are being addressed and notice whether the person patiently makes efforts to answer your questions and provides useful information that helps orient and reassure you.

In an emergency situation, due to time limitations, it may be necessary to get most of your information from an assistant, such as a nurse, medical resident, or physician's assistant. But with all nonemergency procedures, make sure that you meet the actual person who will be working directly with you and take time to form a sense of who they are and how you feel in their presence. This rapport can be an important factor in your healing. Many patients are unnecessarily surprised when they do not meet their surgeon until moments before they are wheeled into the operating room, allowing little or no time for questions and a sense of connection. Be proactive—make sure you have as satisfying and complete an encounter as is possible, given your particular circumstances.

It's generally a good idea to take someone with you to any preparatory meetings. It is not uncommon for patients to become overwhelmed with the information they are being given and flooded by their emotional reactions. An advocate, such as a close friend or family member, can ask additional questions you might not think of in that moment, take notes, or record/transcribe the information presented.

Remember that one of your goals is to try to develop a team of support around you. Ratings, credentials, and recommendations are certainly important, but also pay attention to your gut reactions during your first meeting with a health professional. What is your sense of their competence and integrity? Remember that you are the "customer," and it's your right to get the best fit you can find. If you sense that the professional is not connecting with you and is not present, this can be a warning sign that you may not get the type of attention you need and deserve throughout the process. At that point, you may opt for a second opinion from a different professional.

Cynthia was a successful businesswoman who had been experiencing intermittent abdominal pain for several months. She had experimented with many homeopathic supplements and various treatment programs, including Pilates, yoga, and acupuncture, as well as seeking help from her internist and her gynecologist. On the basis of several inconclusive tests, she was referred to an oncologist due to the possibility of early-stage ovarian cancer.

After further testing, she was sent to a surgeon who had been highly recommended by several friends and treating professionals, including her oncologist. During the meeting, Cynthia noted that the surgeon appeared preoccupied and rushed, barely looked up from the papers on his desk, and was dismissive of some of her questions. When she left his office, she felt discouraged and anxious.

Because of these reactions, Cynthia sought a second opinion from a second surgeon. This one was young, personable, made good contact, and gave Cynthia almost an hour of unhurried time to cover all of her points of concern, adding discussion of in-depth case examples of several of his patients who had similar ovarian findings. This time, when she left this surgeon's office, she felt lighter and more connected.

The next day, however, she realized she had forgotten to ask the more personable surgeon a question about the type of pain medication that would be useful after the surgery. Cynthia also felt anxious about the fact that this doctor was so young, wondering if he had sufficient experience with the type of ovarian surgery she needed. She called his office, and received immediate, reassuring service from his staff. "We understand that there are many important questions to be resolved. Medication is certainly essential for you to be clear about. This will be covered in depth at the appointment to prepare you for surgery, but let's connect you with the doctor's surgical assistant so that you can get started with that discussion now. And if you have questions after your surgery, the doctor will let you know how you can best reach him directly."

Although Cynthia had to weigh the advantages of the extra years of experience and expertise the first surgeon had accumulated, she decided to trust the inner safety she felt with the second. Cynthia also researched the younger doctor online and discovered that his patients gave him high ratings for his skill and care. She commented to one of her friends, "The first guy may be an excellent surgeon, but I don't believe he is a good surgeon for me."

In seeking out other information that can prepare you, strive for a balance of the informal and the scientific. That is, it's fine to solicit information directly from friends or on blog sites, but it is also important to ask for and read any information provided by your doctor. Many medical offices now offer informational packets with photographs and diagrams, checklists for complete preparation procedures, and even video and audio presentations that are very complete and sometimes interactive, offering opportunities to ask common questions and receive complete answers. Take this step seriously. Make sure you are as fully informed as possible without overdoing this effort so that you do not become overwhelmed or exhausted. This is the balance that will support your successful outcome.

Like Cynthia, you may discover that tuning into your felt-sense responses during interviews with experts, reading information about procedures you are considering, or discussing possibilities with friends or loved ones will help you steer toward safety and success. Body sensations connected to fear, such as tightness, constriction, pressure, or heaviness, may alert you to possible unconscious perceptions of danger or threat, while the somatic experiences of expansion, comfort, and openness may suggest safety instead.

We suggest that if you are undergoing major surgery that you find out about follow-up rehabilitation, including what is involved, recommendations for facilities or rehab therapies, and expected duration of rehab treatment, as well as the aftereffects that you can expect. If possible, you may want to make arrangements well in advance, so that you are able to choose the rehab facility that you prefer.

Assembling all of this information is obviously time consuming. You may need to ask for a longer appointment or a second, follow-up appointment to cover everything you want to include. Do not feel apologetic about asking for the help you need. Feel free to ask for the time that you need to feel prepared, and then make sure that you get it. If the doctor or office staff reacts negatively to your requests, this is another red flag that the fit may not be a good one for you.

One of our colleagues conducted a simple survey with a reconstructive surgeon and an anesthesiologist, inquiring about the patients most likely to do well with their procedures. These professionals reported that the patients who asked the most questions and persisted in exploring everything they were concerned with, had doubts about, or felt anxious about, were actually the most cooperative with their medical team. More importantly, these individuals recovered the most rapidly and had the fewest side effects following their surgery. However, if you are the type of individual that would rather "not worry about details," and just leave everything to the surgeon, then less information might be best for you.

WORKING WITH FEAR AND ANXIETY BEFORE YOUR PROCEDURE

It's entirely natural to encounter fears before undergoing any medical procedure, especially surgery. We suggest that you use the tools that you've learned so far in the Freedom from Pain program, especially the breathing methods, to work with the anxiety that tends to build before a medical event. Regardless of which tools you choose, pay particular attention to any specific fears and thoughts, such as "The surgery won't go well and I'll be left with more pain than before" or "I may not come back from this; I might die." Balance these fearful thoughts with the facts about that surgery; for example, 95 percent of many procedures occur without any complications.

When connecting with whatever your fear is, first find the sensations it evokes in your body. These might include tightness, quivering, heaviness, an increase in your usual pain sensations, and so on. Next, you might use circle breathing (see exercise on page 24) to begin shifting these sensations while opening channels of moving energy in your body. Use any variation of circle breathing that works for you.

Other breathing methods you've learned in this program can help in different ways. For example, voo breathing and sounding can help regulate more intense states of fear and panic (see exercise on page 34). You might want to try this now, focusing on a sensation of fear, stress, or pain, and breathing through it using a nice long "voo" sound on your exhale. Notice what happens in your body, especially to the sensations connected with fear. Then become aware of any thoughts that seem associated with the sensations; in particular, notice that they are only thoughts and not true facts.

You can also try different sounds with your breathing. Sounding "ahh," for example, as you exhale, may turn on calming responses that are similar to what happens when you naturally sigh, "Ahhhh . . ." with relief or pleasure. Try this now. Take a breath in, and let it out while sounding "ahh" with a nice open sound. What is this like for you right now?

Many people find that an "ahh" breath automatically helps the body to be relaxed and open. This makes sense, of course, because we say "Ahh" spontaneously when we're relaxed, as though to say, "Thank goodness I'm past that hard time and I can take a breather."

Another approach is to develop steady breathing, where your inhale is about the same length as your exhale. If helpful, when you're breathing in you can count to three or four, and then while breathing out, use the same count. Try this right now if you'd like. What effect does it have? The use of steady breathing may actually help you begin to feel steadier when you anticipate the surgery or procedure.

You may also find that you can use the simple Just One Breath method (see page 33) as you practice being more aware of tension and anxiety and pausing to follow the movement of one in-breath and out-breath through your body. Make sure that you allow the out-breath to extend as slowly and completely as possible.

Whatever breathing or relaxation techniques you're going to use, practice them well in advance of surgery. You don't want to be in a situation on the night before your procedure trying to learn how to do something when you're at your most anxious and vulnerable. If you've practiced ahead, then when you're in an altered state of consciousness, you're more likely to shift automatically into some type of breathing process or regulation technique that has worked.. One way to help this along is to experiment with the mini breathing exercises suggested in the previous few paragraphs. Then, record your results in your pain journal to support your awareness of what is most effective and provide yourself with guidance for further practice.

Other strategies to use with pre-procedure anxiety and fear include the use of *informal states of intensive focus* that have proven helpful in the past. If you've participated in activities such as music or dance performance, public speaking, or athletic events, for example, you've probably felt highly engaged and able to screen out all distractions, including fear and exhaustion, to achieve the focus you want. You might find it very useful to practice applying your natural state of intense positive focus to help develop your expectations of your current medical challenge.

A simple example of positive focus can be found in the experience of Martha, who had endured a long, complicated, and excruciating labor giving birth to her first child. Before the birth of her second child, she practiced imagining the labor process as a series of increasingly difficult climbs in the mountains where she often hiked. Each uphill effort was followed by downhill relief, until the hike culminated in the final push of immense effort to reach the mountaintop. At last she arrived and entered into the wondrous merging of exhaustion and exhilaration. This indeed was how her delivery experience with her second child turned out.

The main idea, no matter what strategy you use, is to stay as active and focused as possible throughout your process, because active engagement allows you to stay in a place of empowerment so that you do not succumb to helplessness, where you feel frozen, like a victim having something done *to* you.

Finally, consider what kinds of positive healing messages or intentions you want to give yourself about healing. Just as fears create constricted imprints on sensations in the body, positive intentions can stimulate more expansive body sensations.

As you get ready for any invasive procedures, ask yourself, "What is truly healing for me?" Each time you ask this question, you may receive a slightly different answer, but if you ask over time during your process of preparation, you will notice patterns that seem to be in alignment with balance and harmony in your entire organism.

Some of your findings about what is truly healing for you also can evolve into specific self-suggestions for healing from the upcoming procedure. Examples of such affirmations are:

- I want to experience optimal healing.
- I want to have only as much swelling and pain as is necessary for complete and optimal recovery.
- I can have complete and rapid recovery knowing that my body will respond exactly in the way that is needed so that this procedure can be completely successful in every way.

Take a moment and say each of these phrases out loud or silently to yourself. Where does each intention live in your body? What sensations does each evoke? Based on your answers, modify your statements further until you find the ones that elicit the most complete sense of resonance, the clearest "yes" response from your body. Note them in your journal so you can use these as part of your preparation practice.[1]

As important as it is to develop your own positive messages for yourself, it can be even more helpful to suggest statements to be used by medical personnel staffing your procedure. Rachel needed to have a particularly invasive kind of colonoscopy, and so she discussed possible problems in advance with her doctor. (In a previous attempt at the surgery, Rachel's ileum had tightened and they had to stop the colonoscopy.) She asked the surgeon to say softly, "Open, ileum" if any tightening occurred again. That evening, after the effects of the anesthesia had cleared, her doctor called to say that the procedure was completely successful because when he said, "Open, ileum," the ileum responded by opening so they could complete the process!

Therefore, we also suggest that you choose several suggestions that you would like to hear during the procedure or surgery—to reinforce when things are going well. We sometimes invite our clients to write these on index cards and give them to surgeons, anesthesiologists, doctors, or nurses—whoever seems most responsive—and ask them to say these out loud during the intervention itself. Some useful suggestions include:

"Everything is going very well."
"Your body is responding in ways that will allow this
      procedure to be complete and successful in every way."
"We are very pleased by what we are seeing."

A final note is that sometimes preparation needs to include supplements that can improve immune functioning after surgery. This is particularly relevant for individuals who have had previous infections. Certain supplements called *immunonutrients* include omega-3 fatty acids and arginine, which may stimulate human growth hormone to promote regrowth and repair of tissues and muscles following surgery. Other possibilities include glutamine to support tissue repair and recovery and amino acids that may help to heal tears. You may want to research the use of nutritional supplements and discuss those as part of your pre-surgical consultation.

MINIMIZING THE IMPACT
OF PREVIOUS TRAUMATIC EVENTS

Another strategy to maximize your success and prevent further emotional and physical trauma is to review what has not gone well for you in the past, in terms of healing and recovery. Many people don't see the importance of connecting with prior traumatic medical events, or may simply have repressed those experiences so that they are inaccessible.

Take a few moments right now to think about even minor previous surgeries, such as dental surgery, stitches to repair open wounds, the process of setting broken bones, and even the experience of receiving painful inoculations as a child. ✑

If you like, you can note your inventory in your pain journal. If you are aware that you have a significant trauma history, or you begin to feel overwhelmed while taking your own inventory, please consider consulting an appropriate psychotherapist. It can be helpful to have support when you review past medical events and your reactions to them.

John was struggling with the decision about whether to have back surgery. He was a superb athlete, but no matter how he tried to create a balanced rehab program following a series of sports injuries, his progress continued to stall, and even to decline. When he thought about why he was so scared of having the recommended surgery, he realized that when he had been ten years old, he had climbed a challenging mountain with his older brother and his friends. Because he wanted to prove that he could keep up with them, he overreached for tree roots to support himself instead of waiting for a rope to be thrown. John fell more than twenty-five feet and landed on his back. His brother took him to the emergency room and he was given stitches and a series of shots.

This was a painful and scary experience and one that he had never told his parents about because he had not gotten their permission to make the climb. As he thought about his current surgical possibility, he realized he was afraid he would "overreach" by attempting more than he could safely handle and that he might put himself in even greater difficulty. As he explored this past event, however, he realized that there were many differences between his past and present situations. Not only was he preparing well in advance, but he had nothing to prove to others. Sorting out the past from the present with professional assistance allowed John to approach surgery with more confidence, and his recovery went very well. It is not uncommon for children to hide accidents from their parents because they have been doing things that they were not (or believed they were not) supposed to do and feared that their parents would be very angry with them.

A helpful question to ask yourself during your review of past medical procedures is: "What was missing back then that might have made all the difference in having a positive outcome?" If your answer is "lack of support," then you'll want to make sure that you secure more than enough support at the present time. If your procedure includes a hospital stay, it is valuable to plan for one or more advocates to be with you throughout the event so that your important needs can be attended to more consistently and medical errors can be prevented. This is a valuable service that friends can provide for each other.

You'll also want to arrange support after the procedure and during your recovery process. If recovery is estimated to last longer than a day or two, you'll want to line up friends, neighbors, and loved ones to bring food, help you negotiate painful activities, especially if you live alone, and provide transportation and companionship for follow-up appointments, including physical therapy and other rehab. It's important to plan ahead for even simple procedures.

Peter recently had a hernia repair and was grateful that there was someone there to take care of simple needs and provide support. He had chosen to have the surgery at an outpatient facility to minimize the risk of contracting an MRSA infection (the serious "superbug" that is found in many hospitals). When he arrived and met the anesthesiologist, Peter was told that it was only possible to use a different anesthetic in this outpatient facility than the one he had chosen with his surgeon. Although first alarmed, Peter was, with the support of an accompanying friend, able to calmly change his previously well-planned decision. Without this support, he might have been unduly frightened.

If you find yourself feeling unmotivated and stuck (in terms of arranging care for yourself), think of someone in your community who has been through a similar medical procedure and might coach you through it. Loved ones are usually pleased to contribute their own learning to help you master the challenges you face.

Some people have difficulty with this step, believing they are imposing further on family or friends who have already given significant support and assistance. If you notice that you are not reaching out to make secure arrangements for your care, it's a good idea to negotiate the help you need. For example, you can offer a trade or an exchange of in-kind support once you have recovered. Whatever your gifts, whether cooking, sewing, coaching, accounting, or tutoring, you can find a good way to return favors so that your relationships remain comfortably in balance. One of Maggie's friends thanked all members of her social community who provided food and other forms of assistance during her recovery from hip replacement surgery with a celebratory dance party.

It might be a good idea to use your pain journal to note what you think you will need during your recovery process, as well as a list of people or organizations that might help you.

CREATING A PAIN PLAN
FOR YOUR MEDICAL PROCEDURE

When creating a plan to regulate and manage your pain before, during, and after any medical procedure, be sure to consider your whole self and the totality of your pain needs, no matter how demanding or eccentric they may seem. Keep in mind that your overall intention is to accept and respond to yourself in such a way that your body feels safe enough to heal completely. Unmanaged pain is not in alignment with these goals.

Make sure that you discuss with your prescribing professional your known needs for medication.[2] Emphasize your need for a *secure* pain plan that you can trust so that you can focus on healing. Discuss past experiences that might influence current choices of medication or anesthesia, especially experiences when you were under-medicated or had adverse reactions to medications that were used. If you are hypersensitive to most medications, be direct about this and arrange for an approach that follows the principle, "Start low and go slow"—that is, it may be best to try any medication at a low dose with careful monitoring and orders for flexible increases or alternatives, depending on your moment-to-moment responses.

It is especially important *not* to have gaps in your medication during recovery. It is amazing how many people are sent home or to a rehab facility following surgery without proper pain medications. Make sure that you are not one of them! Find out who the "go to" person for medication is on your medical team, and discuss your needs at length until you feel secure. Know the options and the precise process for making decisions if your pain unexpectedly increases at any time before, during, and after the procedure.

Do not accept the assertion that you'll be able to discuss your pain needs during your postoperative or follow-up appointment with your doctor. Many patients have been blindsided by changes in the medical professional's schedule that leave them without timely access to refills or alternatives to medications that aren't working properly. *Insist* on reliable access to your doctor or prescribing professional—this can include their cell phone number.

Remember, although addiction to pain medication is a potential concern, it is much more dangerous to get behind on pain regulation since this can set up an overwhelming situation that prevents healing. Instead, when pain is properly controlled, the likelihood for addiction is greatly reduced. Also remember, unpleasant side effects are a reasonable compromise when it comes to effective pain management.

A common, unmanaged pain situation happens when the patient is not sleeping well enough to heal and recover, or when the pain remains at an 8, 9, or 10 (on a 10–point pain scale) such that it is virtually intolerable, and prevents the patient from optimal participation in physical therapy and other recovery activities. *Make sure* that an appropriate medical professional is willing and available to monitor your pain situation carefully enough to prevent these complications and to help you transition at the right time to different doses or different medications that will help you stay regulated.

Zina's Pain Plan

Zina had planned a hip replacement surgery to coincide with her sister's visit from Ireland so that she would have help during the first two weeks of her recovery. Since she had talked to friends at length who had had the same procedure, she became aware both of the factors that make recovery difficult as well as the resources that contribute to success.

She insisted on an hour-long meeting with her surgeon and told him about her current use of medications, which included ibuprofen and Percocet for breakthrough pain. The surgeon agreed that Zina should remain on these medications through the time of her surgery, so that she would remain stable.

Zina also told him that in the past, following a prior shoulder surgery, she had not done well with either morphine or codeine. Her surgeon reassured her that fentanyl (from another class of opiates) would provide similar pain relief immediately after surgery. He also told her that she would take home a prescription for additional pain medication that would help her taper off of the fentanyl. Zina made sure to arrange for patient-controlled administration of the medication, which occurred by pressing a button. Her surgeon asked her to check in with his assistant one week following the surgery to discuss how her medications were performing. Furthermore, he emphasized to Zina that if she was not responding well to the medication before the follow-up visit, she was to call his assistant immediately, who would then get in touch with him.

Because of this secure pain plan, there were no gaps in Zina's pain treatment and she was able to make steady progress, sleep well, and respond well to physical therapy in a rehab facility. One month following the surgery, she was off of all medications except for ibuprofen with a low dose of Vicodin for breakthrough pain, which she used once or twice per week.

Most hospitals and many medical providers now include a patient's right to pain management as part of any treatment plan. It might be helpful for you to review and discuss with your medical team "The Pain Patient Bill of Rights" published by the National Pain Foundation (nationalpainfoundation.org), or other similar guidelines prior to your procedure.[3]

SPECIAL ISSUES IN PREVENTING TRAUMA

There are several issues related to the topics in this chapter that deserve special attention.

Making Good Decisions

It is helpful for you to think about appropriate steps in the process of making good decisions about whether or not to have surgery or other medical procedures. Although no one can guarantee your success, if you are well informed and have taken the time to think through all of the essential questions, you are less likely to experience unpleasant surprises that can trigger traumatic reactions and/or reduced healing during and after medical events.

If you are deciding to have surgery because you want to secure a life that is freer from pain, we remind you that it's important to understand that you may not get rid of all of the pain, and in some cases may end up with more pain. This may, in part, be because the surgery does not really address the underlying cause of pain. This is one reason why we strongly suggest that you seek a second opinion, address possible psychological factors with a therapist, as well as use the various exercises in this program. Also, any surgery is invasive to some extent and to some degree causes trauma and scar tissue. This can result in more pain later on. Some scar tissue can be reduced through acupuncture and special massage techniques. This should be done only after healing is complete.

No surgery, not even a minor one, is risk-free. To decide if a procedure is right for you, learn as much as possible about it, including its possible benefits and *risks*. Patients who know the facts about surgery and other treatments can better work with their doctors to make decisions based on science as well as on patient preferences.[4]

Here are some questions you may want to ask your doctor or surgeon during your decision process. You can note your questions and your doctors' answers in your pain journal. Also it is generally advisable to have a calm, centered friend or relative with you. Often we forget important information because we are, understandably, stressed.

Do I really need this surgery or procedure? Is there some other way to treat my condition? What are the alternatives and what are the risks and benefits of each?

What will happen if I wait until later to have surgery? Or never have it at all?

How often does this type of surgery really help my kind of problem? How much does it help? (This information comes from outcome studies. Indeed, when outcome studies have been carried out, some common back and knee surgeries, for example, have been shown to be ineffectual.)

Does the doctor, surgeon, hospital, or surgery center have extensive experience with this kind of procedure? What is the range of outcomes the professional has witnessed? Here is a brief "check-list" for you to follow.

- Is the surgeon experienced and qualified to perform the surgery? How many times has he or she done this procedure? You can also check on the Internet to see if they've been sued for malpractice.
- What complications or side effects might I have?
- What kind of pain might I have? How will it be treated?
- How long will it take me to recover? Will I need help at home? If so, what kind of help might I need and what are the best ways to go about receiving this kind of help?
- How can I best prevent unpleasant surprises in terms of billing and insurance?

Coping with Repeated Injury and Trauma

There is heightened awareness these days of what is called cumulative trauma disorder (CTD) and Repetitive Stress Injury, which can result from repetitive movement and overuse of various parts of the body. One such example is carpal tunnel syndrome.

It's always preferable in these cases to explore more conservative, nonsurgical treatments first in order to relieve discomfort from overuse. Splints may be recommended as an early treatment to protect and rest sore areas. Anti-inflammatory medicines are often prescribed along with physical therapy, as well as ice packs,[5] acupuncture, ultrasound, or electrical stimulation. Your doctor or physical therapist may suggest special exercises that can help tissues move safely while they heal.

You may need help evaluating both your work (especially computer typing) and recreational activities to determine how they are adding to your problem. Keep in mind that unrelieved tension resulting from stress and further injury restricts the flow of blood, causing muscles and nerves to receive inadequate oxygen and nutrients, which aggravates the symptoms of CTD. Resting the injured area during work and play activities can relieve tension and allow for more complete recovery.

Well-trained physical therapists, physiatrists, and osteopaths, as well as practitioners of awareness-based exercise programs like Feldenkrais, Pilates, and the Alexander technique, may be able to help you achieve better posture and spinal alignment. They can also teach you ways of bending, balancing, and moving that support recovery from injury (including stretches), as well as help you modify your work or other environments to prevent re-injury.

Playing It Safe with Ongoing Medication

Sometimes it will be necessary to take medications over an extended time period in order to regulate your pain adequately. If this is the case, you will need to give your entire health care team adequate information so they can help you use your medications effectively. Tell them about:

- all prescription medications
- over-the-counter medications
- vitamins, minerals, and all dietary supplements

You will also need to enlist their help in properly tapering off medications to avoid negative side effects, prevent recurrence of negative reactions to medications (or to supplements), or evaluate interactions between different medications used for different medical issues in addition to pain. Particularly, there are several common supplements that interfere with blood clotting. This can be critical information. These include fish oils, garlic extract, ginkgo biloba, and even certain (protein) digestive enzymes.

It is sometimes tempting to serve as your own doctor, especially when you have to wait to see a specialist or other provider. A far safer route is to talk to your pharmacist instead of depending on your own assessment if you have questions about your medication situation. Otherwise, write down important questions when you do have a meeting with your pain doctor, making a list of all prescriptions, medications, and supplements (including the dosage strength and frequency of dosage for each one).

Make sure to take this information with you to all appointments. Also, find a reliable way to keep track of all your medications so that you take them as prescribed. Some people use a pillbox while others use tracking methods such as a schedule with check-off spaces for daily a.m. and p.m. doses. Ask for help when you are having difficulty sticking with your medication plan. And above all, make sure you involve others so that you have access to more than just your own feedback.

It is important to *over-prepare* for pain and anxiety. We often coach people to work out a pain plan with their medical professionals, well ahead of the date of the medical procedures, so that they feel secure. For many people, having a prescription for a few doses of a strong narcotic can serve as a good insurance policy; you know it is there *if* you need it. This sense of security, in itself, can decrease the experience of anxiety and pain. We've found that patients often choose not to use this type of medication, or will use it judiciously, since they feel secure with the resources and other medications they have. This ounce of preparation is easily worth the proverbial pound of cure. And, of course, should pain arise, you have already learned and practiced many techniques for dealing with it. But remember, do not be afraid to use a narcotic if the pain is beginning to rise sharply—providing your doctor is in agreement.

In our next and final chapter, we will take you further along your journey out of pain to the third stage, resilience and continued recovery. The skills involved in this final stage not only give you the edge on pain, but are also the tools that support the vibrant and focused life that you deserve to live.

CHAPTER SEVEN

Resilience, Continued Recovery, and Restoring the Deep Self

*Paradoxically, we achieve true wholeness only by embracing
our fragility and sometimes, our brokenness.*
—JALAJA BONHEIM, *APHRODITE'S DAUGHTERS*

AS WE HAVE EMPHASIZED throughout this program, how we respond to threat and the high activation of our nervous system will determine whether we will clear the impact of the threat and even become stronger from it. The answers lie in the unspoken, automatic mechanisms of our body and nervous system. We all possess these resources, but we must learn how to access them, and more importantly, how not to interfere with them. This is the third stage, resilience and continued recovery to restore the deep self. We'll discuss each aspect of this stage separately: resilience, continued recovery, and the process of restoring the balance and strength of the deep self.

RESILIENCE

Resilience is defined as the dynamic process that allows us to exhibit positive responses when confronted with adversity, trauma, tragedy, threats, or significant sources of stress. Resilience is variable across situations—that is, individuals who demonstrate competence and the ability to adapt in some areas of risk may show problems in other areas. For example, it's common for some people to be more resilient in dealing with workplace adversity while indicating deficits in resilience with personal and family relationships.

Resilience is enhanced in the process of exploring body experience. There are important ways that we can learn to encourage the discovery of resilience, so essential to healing pain.

Healing Through the Body

The key to healing pain, as you have been learning, lies in understanding and working with body reactions. By cultivating body awareness and maintaining sensation-based focus, we learn to befriend these trauma-based sensations and then to move through them. Since people struggling with pain and trauma often perceive their bodies as the enemy, this "befriending" is a key capacity—a capacity which also provides the opportunity for ongoing vibrancy.

Embodiment creates connection and reduces the need for dissociation and escaping from the body. Overcoming the need to dissociate from the body allows us to learn to feel what the body is feeling. With this connection, we move toward enhanced mind-body-heart-spirit awareness, and the possibility of wholeness.

How Curiosity Saved the Cat and Can Help You Too

We have emphasized throughout this program the importance of opening the door to curiosity. Recall a time when you were really excited and curious about something. What is going on in your body right now as you experience this recollection?

Once you open the door to curiosity, exploration, and connection with body experience, you've already made a very big step in transforming trauma. Curiosity about your body also helps to turn off the trauma alarm system. Then it becomes possible to retrieve and evaluate information from your body using your curious, open mind and its skills in tracking sensations, making cognitive and emotional connections, and arriving at symbolic meaning.[1]

Reaping Your Just Rewards

It is also helpful to discover reward systems that may be in place for you and to understand how these reward systems operate and can be changed so that you can learn to feel more pleasure. An example is Rebecca, who had spina bifida and significant early trauma, including pre-birth difficulties, multiple developmental challenges, and a traumatizing surgery. As is true for many people who have trauma, we discovered that her major reward system was based on *avoidance.* She largely avoided uncomfortable feelings, including shame about her physical limitations and the way her body looked. Escape was her default "reward."

It was a major breakthrough for Rebecca to realize that when she became fully present while tracking her body experience or during her practice of mindfulness, the newly discovered feelings were much more rewarding. The felt sense was a far better reward to work toward, and more likely to connect her with resilience and positive feelings.

Daniel, a depressed young man with chronic neck, back, and shoulder pain from years of computer programming, found that his reward system was to avoid criticism and judgment from his boss. In learning to focus on the reward of approaching what he wanted to experience instead, which was the freedom to be creative and the confidence to express his creativity at work, Daniel discovered feelings of triumph and well-being.

What about you? Pause and think for a few moments about the rewards that motivate you most. Do they center on avoidance? What about the pursuit of ease and pleasure? How might you make a shift to pursue ease and pleasure in your life today? You might want to make this a day for journaling about new possibilities for rewards to follow and encourage change in this direction. If you choose to do so, what do you discover? ✑

Mindfulness and Resilience

We encourage you to strengthen your resilience by serving as a midwife, mindful witness, and coach for your own healing process. There is now excellent research on the neurobiology of mindfulness and other specific skill-based approaches and how they can help boost resilience.

Dr. Jon Kabat-Zinn, considered to be one of the foremost proponents of mindfulness, has studied the long-term effects of his mindfulness-based stress reduction program, which is offered in many hospitals and through many organizations around the world. Among other results, research shows that after mindfulness training, there's an increased activity in the left frontal lobe.[2]

Somatic Experiencing, the bedrock of the Freedom from Pain program, is an approach that teaches intensive mindfulness of body experience. It's important to know that developing the skills of focused attention, awareness, and curiosity may be linked to positive changes in the brain. In short, these experiences become a more rewarding experience for the individual.

One effective way of connecting with your resilience is through the energy of positive intentions. Although affirmations have long been used to enhance healing, only recently have they been used to connect with the body (See page 112 for more about affirmations).[3]

EXERCISE: Resilience and Positive Intentions

We invite you now to think of several intentions you want to affirm at this point in your healing process. Practice saying each one out loud and connect in your body with the energy of that statement:

- My body is more and more my friend in healing
  my pain.
- As I inhabit my body in more ways and more of the
  time, I'm getting to know who I am in my deepest self.
- I am more confident that I can use the tools from this
  program to help myself move out of pain.
- I am trusting other people more and believe I have
  something to share with them.
- I find myself more able to respond with open sexuality
  when I'm intimate with my partner.

Where do each of these statements "live" in your body? As you connect
with their energy, how can you use one or more of them to connect with
an overall sense of resilience?

Write about your experience with this exercise in your pain journal.

It's important that the wording of affirmations reflects where you are in
your pain journey as well as where you are headed. Michelle, for example,
found the best results with the phrase: "Even though I get discouraged
and depressed, I am still in a better place with my pain than I was three
months ago." After she became comfortable with the positive effects of
this affirmation, she shifted to: "Sometimes I forget how much progress
I've made, so I'm learning to focus on little sensations of pleasure."

From a mindfulness point of view, it is best to begin by affirming
your acceptance of what *is,* as well as what is *beginning* to change, and
hopefully will continue to change.

Joy and Triumph

How does the Freedom from Pain model lead to joy? How can we help
to orchestrate experiences that lead to joy and triumph? First, it's important to realize that on the other side of trauma is triumph. When we
master our traumas and are able to free the energies bound in the fight,

flight, or freeze response, the lightness or freedom of being emerges as our natural state.

EXERCISE: Experiencing Triumph

Think about some of the peak moments of your life. Maybe they were related to physical achievements such as climbing mountains or completing a marathon or cross-country bicycle trip. Or perhaps they were connected with awards for academic achievements or recognition of a talent or skill.

Find and feel the moment of triumph. If you are distracted by details and thoughts, bring your focus back to the sensations of that triumphant experience. Keep coming back to the triumphant moment. Whatever the occasion, *how* does it feel in your body right now? What, for example, do you notice in your chest and in your spine?

Now find a moment of triumph in freeing yourself from pain. Maybe it was receiving the positive results of an X-ray or an MRI or completing the first week when your pain levels stayed low consistently between 0 and 4. Maybe you can recall yourself saying, "I never thought I'd be able to do that again and now I can!" Wherever and whenever you find this triumph over pain inside, feel it, embrace it, and cherish the sensations of triumph in your body.

Taking your time, track these sensations through your feet and legs, your core and belly, your chest and shoulders, your neck and head, hands and arms. As you feel these sensations extending and moving through your body, where do you find the center of expansion, aliveness, and triumph? How can you place a bookmark in your mind's eye so that you can find this moment again? Can you imagine using it as an antidote to discouragement as your recovery from pain continues?

Write about your experience with this exercise in your pain journal.

The Skill of Titration

In chemistry, in order to combine potentially dangerous compounds (for example hydrochloric acid and caustic soda or lye), one must place a single drop from one substance into another, never combining them all at once since doing so would cause a violent explosion. When, in contrast, a single drop of either compound is added to a container of the other, the result might be something like an Alka-Seltzer fizzle—just a little bit of a discharge. Gradually, this process transforms the two corrosive substances into salt and water, not only benign, but the basic building blocks of life.

Because trauma-related sensations can be so intense, we need to explore them one drop at a time. Each time, for example, we might experience a little shaking and trembling, or a small movement that might warm the coldness of the body. Perhaps we will feel some lifting of corrosive shame, or a tender feeling long forgotten. Then we wait. We let the sensations settle before engaging the next cycle of activation and discharge.

An example of this is our work with Thomas. Thomas complained of feeling angry about almost everything in his life, including a severe car accident that left him with serious, unrelenting neck and shoulder pain. After his return to work, he was passed over for several promotions, his girlfriend broke up with him, and his family relationships were tenuous. His early trauma history included ongoing physical abuse by his alcoholic father.

When Thomas began to talk about these difficulties, his hands automatically tightened into fists. Encouraged to feel the energy held in his fists, Thomas commented, "I'd like to punch out that boss of mine who won't give me a break!" We encouraged him to *imagine* punching movements and tell us what he experienced. "My arms feel strong and they want to move and really hit something; mostly, I feel my power."

The next step was to guide him in allowing his arms to move forward in slow motion. His tendency, like those of many people who try this technique, was to want to make rapid, jerky motions with his arms and fists. We suggested instead that he move more slowly and easily. Thomas began to let his right arm slowly move toward the imagined target of his boss's face. Using the techniques explored in chapter 5 (page 97), we held a pillow in front of Thomas so he could direct his anger at it.

After his movements settled, he looked calmer and more focused. "I know now," he reflected, "that I can stand up for myself; I don't need to be a victim." When he connected more completely with his right fist, he said, "That's surprising. I thought the best feeling would be to smash his face with my fists. Actually, what's feeling best right now is that I have a right to explain my position to him. My whole body seems to relax more, and I can feel a letting go through my neck and shoulder."

What resulted for Thomas was a slow, gradual transformation, without any "explosion," that allowed natural resilient energy to emerge. This is the heart of the second phase of ongoing transformation discussed in chapter 4, and also serves as the momentum for the third stage as well.

The Rhythms of Resiliency

Staying curious about what you do or say helps to lead to that path of transformation. It's important that you find your own rhythm that moves slowly enough so that you can follow the imprint of trauma in the body as well as the wellspring of your resiliency.

When finding your own natural rhythms, you'll notice that you are naturally pendulating back and forth. The practice of pendulation allows you to begin to tap into those innate rhythms. This shift allows movement through the rhythms of resilience, which can become like a dance. You will then naturally shift between present moment, past history, and future possibility. You might want to note these shifts in your journal as part of tracking your progress through this program.

Recovery of the Deep Self

Recovery of the deep self is intimately connected to the experience of resilience. We have worked with many individuals who have lived through horrifyingly painful experiences, including survivors of the

Holocaust and other forms of torture, victims of many kinds of abuse and domestic violence, and those who have suffered extreme loss.

We are moved in our encounters with people in these situations by the numerous ways that the body has been able to rebound and continue on with life, as well as how the flickering flame of the deep self can reignite, when given opportunities for careful, calibrated support. The *recovery* of some sense that we have a deep self,[4] uncontaminated by trauma, pain, or adversity, is an initial step in its enduring *restoration*. In the final section of this chapter we will address this deep transformation.

Challenges to Further Recovery

The path to recovery has several common pitfalls that can interfere with transformation and the emergence of the deep self. It's important to identify and prepare for these well in advance so that you are not blindsided, as this can impede recovery.

1. Recovery involves reconnection with some difficult
   emotions, particularly fear, anger, rage, and shame.
   The challenge is not to get stuck in these strong
   emotions, but to learn to connect with, and move
   through them, as you witnessed in Thomas's work
   with his anger.

   Often, when you are threatened or traumatized,
   you experience a wave of rage, which is a self-protective
   response related to the fight response. We don't realize
   that this is something that is *moving through* us. Instead,
   we get caught in the anger, either by trying to suppress
   it or by acting out the rage.

   Different therapies tend to encourage these two
   resolutions. The cognitive therapies emphasize getting control of anger, and emotion-based therapies
   emphasize expressing the anger or releasing it. We are

suggesting a third way: embodying the feeling and allowing tracked sensations to move through the body.

When you begin to thaw from the freeze response and shift into intense, challenging emotions related to the fight-and-flight response, it is important to reassure and remind yourself with compassion, "I know this is really scary." You may doubt that you can ever find positive or even neutral feelings. However, there are many ways to support yourself so that this doesn't feel so overwhelming.

2. It is important to connect and reconnect with others. This occurs through the ventral vagal system that is activated in healing relationships with those who support you, as well as with therapy professionals you might be working with. It is essential that you know how you can feel a secure connection in a given moment, and that you can notice where in your body you feel that secure connection.

   Part of ongoing recovery is to stay with your responses rather than rushing in to "try to fix" them or rescue yourself from immediate despair. If this phase is rushed, your emerging connections to relational responses can be interrupted and positive energy that emerges naturally can be lost.

   When you are struggling with unresolved trauma and pain, you may not understand the concept of resiliency. You may confuse recovery with spiritual concepts of the benefits of pain, such as the "no pain, no gain" belief. Instead, it is important to be open to new experiences because they will naturally carry you into resilient recovery.

Since pain is about the loss of connections—with body, community, spirit, family and loved ones—healing pain is about restoring those connections. What is powerfully healing is to create an experience of ongoing recovery that you can identify through your own language and body experiences. Then you can tell yourself, "I just demonstrated the power of resilience." It may be helpful at that point to bring to your awareness some other examples of resilience in your recovery that you have experienced, because then you can anchor past moments of triumph to current experience.

3.   It's also important to remember that resilient recovery is a process. We must keep learning how to find moments of recovery, much like learning meditation or mindfulness. It may help you to understand that recovery is not a specific state that can be sustained over time. People who do not understand this truth often try to cling to moments when recovery from pain is going well, feeling despair when the experience doesn't last indefinitely. Remember that *all* of recovery is a process.

We emphasize that we want you to practice looking for positive movement in one moment of full presence in the "now." Often you can enter the "now" by exploring simple body movements. For example, if you begin moving both hands spontaneously, the left hand might be moving palm up and the right hand might exhibit a downward pushing movement.

Rather than analyzing or interpreting that movement, we encourage you to explore the felt sense of spontaneous movements. What might emerge in this case is a sense that the right hand is pushing away, as an expression of the fight or flight response, or as a combination of defensive and protective movements. You may come to understand that the hand is pushing away something unwanted and is also pushing back, trying to move out of the danger zone.

The other uplifted hand might express a readiness to receive, a longing for help and support. If you're willing to work with both of those hand responses, this can help promote wholeness and integration. In other words, we want you to create inner containment by learning to sit with the entire range of your body responses. This allows you to be more fully alive in any given moment. And aliveness leads, of course, to feelings of joy, vitality, and triumph.

RESTORING THE DEEP SELF

Trauma can be considered the fourth pathway to awakening, the other three being meditation, sex, and death.[5] When we are released from the trauma of pain and past events, we recover our full instincts and the energies that have been trapped in the prison of constriction and collapse. Recovery from trauma means rediscovery of the missing parts of our being that allow us to feel whole and complete, or maybe discovery for the very first time. Then, we can begin to come alive and thrive, finding freedom from the pain of brokenness.

It is this sense of vital aliveness that gifts us with the enduring restoration of wholeness and a sustaining connection with our deep self. Even though we have suffered, and will most certainly suffer again, we can trust our inner knowing and our embodied experience. Given the right tools and the confidence to use them, unnecessary (self-inflicted) suffering becomes just that—unnecessary.

Acknowledgments

From Peter A. Levine

I thank various colleagues, physical therapists, body workers, and a surgeon or two along the way, who have helped me maintain an effective level of functioning and a relatively pain-free life into my seventieth year.

Much appreciation for my parents and brothers who, in so many ways, have encouraged me to take the path that led me toward discovering the human spirit's potent ability to transform suffering. Both my brothers have influenced my thinking about pain. Robert has helped me appreciate the functional route of pain control through his mastery of Traditional Chinese Medicine. Jon conducted the landmark study which revealed the existence of the placebo response mechanism and its role in the brain and body's internal pain regulating system. His pioneering work has been an inspiration, opening a whole new arena of mind-body medicine.

Appreciation to the many animals, both wild and domestic, who have shared their vitality and pure *joie de vivre* with me and who have taught me lessons of self-regulation and resilience.

Finally, I wish to give my deepest recognition and appreciation to the thousands of individual clients I have seen over the past forty years. Their courage has been my greatest teacher and the inspiration for writing this book. Thanks to everyone who has used my books and

Acknowledgments

learning programs, granting me the personal blessing of being able to make a difference in this world.

From Maggie Phillips

One of the greatest challenges we encounter in life is pain. At full force, pain is both indescribable and unmanageable, and isolates us unmercifully from the healing power of having a connection with one another.

I am grateful to the many clients who, during more than thirty-five years of clinical practice, have helped me expand my understanding of the contours of pain and how we best heal. Each of you has strengthened my faith in the unique power of the human spirit to transform even the most unimaginable suffering. I also acknowledge the many colleagues who have helped shape my work and who graciously add their own innovations to extend its effectiveness.

I have been blessed with many spiritual mentors, teachers, and companions—saints and sages from all traditions. I give an especially big, grateful hug to Brother David Steindl-Rast who has taught me so much about the power of divine healing and the art of spiritual life.

I express deep appreciation to my parents and brother who have guided many of the life steps that have led me to the discovery of bright light within the dark prisons of adversity. My thanks also to my extended family of loved ones and friends who have supported, held, inspired, and loved me throughout various life journeys. All of you have taught me well and contribute to all that I teach in the world.

Finally I want to honor Andrea Bryck whose loving patience and endless humor form the compass through each day's complexity, and our dog Casey who tirelessly herds us home.

Together we all make a powerful difference in the world.

Notes

Introduction

1. "Chronic Pain in America: Roadblocks to Relief," a study conducted by Roper Starch Worldwide for American Academy of Pain Medicine, American Pain Society and Janssen Pharmaceutica, (1999).

2. Institute of Medicine, "Relieving Pain in America: A Blueprint for Transforming, Prevention, Care, Education, and Research," The National Academies Press (2011), healthland.time.com/2011/06/29/report-chronic-undertreated-pain-affects-116-million-americans/print/.

3. "Chronic Pain in America."

4. Gallup Organization, "Pain in America: A Research Report," survey conducted for Merck (2000).

5. Institute of Medicine report, "Relieving Pain in America."

6. R. S. Roth, M. E. Geisser, and R. Bates, "The Relation of Post-Traumatic Stress Symptoms to Depression and Pain in Patients with Accident-Related Chronic Pain," *Journal of Pain* 9 (2008): 588–96.

7. For a free, downloadable pain journal and a pain tracking device, please visit reversingchronicpain.com/journal.html and reversingchronicpain.com/tracker.html.

Notes

Chapter 1: Why We Hurt and How We Suffer

1. Eugene Gendlin, *Focusing* (New York: Bantam Books, 1982). This is a classic book that can teach you a great deal about how to focus on your body experience.
2. If massage seems beyond your budget, consider contacting local massage schools in your area. Most massage schools offer low-cost referrals to their student practitioners, who are supervised by instructors and are usually well-trained and eager to please.
3. For additional examples of the language of sensation and tips on how to use it, please visit larisakoehn.com/sensations-list/.

Chapter 2: The Pain Trap

1. Ronald Melzack and Patrick Wall, *The Challenge of Pain* (New York: Penguin, 1996).
2. For more information on circle breathing, see Maggie Phillips, *Reversing Chronic Pain: A 10-Point All-Natural Plan for Lasting Relief* (Berkeley, CA: North Atlantic Books, 2007), 22, and her online program at reversingchronicpain.com.

Chapter 3: Neutralizing the Factors That Cause Chronic Pain

1. Body scans were made popular by Dr. Jon Kabat-Zinn, one of the pioneers in the mindfulness movement. The purpose is to train your focus systematically on various parts of the body while remaining mindful and accepting of any sensations encountered. For more information, please see "Body Scan" in the resources section.
2. This technique is modified from that presented by Neil Fiore, author of *Awaken Your Strongest Self* (New York: McGraw-Hill, 2010).
3. Procedural or implicit memory is a form of long-term memory. Every day, we rely on procedural memory, which allows us to perform simple tasks like tying our shoes or brushing our teeth without consciously thinking about these activities. For more information about how trauma is related to implicit memory

and how Somatic Experiencing can work with procedural or "body" memories, see traumahealing.com/somatic-experiencing/techniques-to-work-through-and-treat-trauma-memory.html.

4. Cortisol is a steroid hormone, or glucocorticoid, produced by the adrenal gland. It is released in response to stress. Most people with PTSD show a low secretion of cortisol and high secretion of catecholamines in their urine in contrast with individuals who demonstrate normal fight and flight responses, when both catecholamine and cortisol levels are elevated. See N. Bohnen, N. Nicolson, J. Sulon, K. Jolles, "Coping Style, Trait Anxiety and Cortisol Reactivity during Mental Stress," *Journal of Psychosomatic Research*, 35(2–3) (1991): 141–47.

5. This study was conducted by Ulrich Sachesse, Susanne von der Heyde, and Gerald Huether, "Stress Regulation and Self-Mutilation," *American Journal of Psychiatry* 159 (April 2002): 672.

6. Dr. Martin Seligman pioneered work in this area and first developed the theory of learned helplessness to help explain situations where humans and other animals have learned to behave helplessly, even when the opportunity is restored to avoid an unpleasant or harmful circumstance to which it has been subjected. "Learned helplessness theory is the view that clinical depression and related mental illnesses may result from a perceived absence of control over the outcome of a situation." (en.wikipedia.org/wiki/Learned_helplessness). See also Martin Seligman, *Helplessness: On Depression, Development, and Death* (San Francisco: W. H. Freeman, 1975). Dr. Seligman has developed the Positive Psychology Center at the University of Pennsylvania, and his work on learned optimism and positive psychology is also of interest in repairing helplessness (see ppc.sas.upenn.edu/publications.htm for selected articles and video on this topic).

7. Robert Scaer, *The Trauma Spectrum: Hidden Wounds and Hidden Resiliency* (New York: W. W. Norton, 2005).

8. Conflict-free imagery has been used to contain or work with conflict-free experience or energy. To learn more about this technique, see Maggie Phillips, *Finding the Energy to Heal: How EMDR, Hypnosis, TFT, Imagery, and Body-Focused Therapy Help Restore Mindbody Health* (New York: W. W. Norton, 2000).

9. The over-energy correction (Cook's Hookup) is very helpful as a stress reduction technique and is also useful in reducing symptoms of anxiety, sleep disturbance, insomnia, and panic. Please see "Energy Approaches" in the resources section for more information and a diagram.

Chapter 4: The Journey Back from Unmanageable Pain

1. The gate theory of pain was introduced by Drs. Ron Melzack and Patrick Hall in 1965 with the finding that special nerve cells (nociceptors) carry nerve signals from the site of injury to the dorsal horn in the back of the spinal cord. Past experience, current experience, and certain psychological factors can shut the gate, inhibiting transmission to the brain, or open the gate to send pain signals directly to the brain. For more information on the gate theory, see Ron Melzack and Patrick Hall, *The Challenge of Pain* (New York: Penguin, 1996), and Maggie Phillips, *Reversing Chronic Pain*.

2. There has been an explosion of pain technology and methodology in recent years. Specific examples of these are described in more detail in the resources section.

3. Increasing concern about addiction to pain drugs makes it harder for professionals to prescribe and harder for people in pain to consider taking certain medications, especially opiates. Research shows that 3–16 percent of people who suffer from chronic pain and are treated with long-term opiate narcotics have a risk of developing addiction to these drugs. There is a much higher percentage (more than 80 percent of this group), however, that does not develop addiction and really benefits from the use of opiates. Consider consulting a doctor

who specializes in pain medicine rather than a general practitioner or a psychiatrist if this is an issue for you. See medicinenet.com/script/main/art.asp?articlekey=50318 for more information.

4. Levine, *In an Unspoken Voice,* 271.

5. Other types of tapping used with pain include energy tapping and bilateral tapping. Energy tapping refers in general to tapping on acupoints in a prescribed sequence to treat many common issues, including anxiety, phobias, pain, and PTSD. The most popular of these is Emotional Freedom Technique (EFT), developed by Gary Craig (visit eftuniverse.com for more information). Tapping has also been used in EMDR (eye movement desensitization and reprocessing) to activate bilateral stimulation. One popular method is the self-help approach developed by Laurel Parnell, *Tapping In: A Step-by-Step Guide to Activating Your Healing Resources through Bilateral Stimulation* (Boulder, CO: Sounds True, 2008).

6. To learn more about inner conflict, see Maggie Phillips and Claire Frederick, *Healing the Divided Self: Clinical and Ericksonian Hypnotherapy for Dissociative Conditions* (New York: W. W. Norton, 1995).

7. Resonance circuits are beyond the scope of this book. Daniel Siegel explores them in *The Mindful Brain: Reflection and Attunement in the Cultivation of Well-Being* (New York: W. W. Norton, 2007).

8. For more information on Brother David and his ministry, see David Steindl-Rast, *Gratefulness, the Heart of Prayer: An Approach to Life in Fullness* (Ramsey, NJ: Paulist Press, 1984), and gratefulness.org.

9. The Institute of HeartMath has published an excellent free e-book on its scientific research called *Science of the Heart: Exploring the Role of the Heart in Human Performance.* This can be downloaded at heartmath.org/research/science-of-the-heart/introduction.html. Another helpful reference is Doc Childre and Howard Martin, *The HeartMath Solution: The Institute of HeartMath's Revolutionary Program for Engaging the Power of the Heart's Intelligence* (New York:

HarperCollins, 1999), which can be ordered at store.heartmath.org/
books/heartmath-solution.

10. This practice is designed to develop Quick Coherence®, which can be
downloaded as a narrative and as an MP3 audio at heartmath.org/
free-services/tools-for-well-being/quick-coherence-adult.html.

11. This meditation is based on one developed by Christopher Germer,
*The Mindful Path to Self-Compassion: Freeing Yourself from Destructive
Thoughts and Emotions* (New York: Guilford Press, 2009). You can
find free downloads and other information at mindfulselfcompassion.
org. Another good source is Sharon Salzberg, *Lovingkindness: The
Revolutionary Art of Happiness* (New York: Shambhala, 2002).

12. Brain plasticity, also called neuroplasticity, is a term used to describe
the brain's ability to change at any age due to new experience. This
new science replaces the previous theory that DNA and genetics
predetermined an individual's developmental history, including health,
personality, and other attributes. For more information, also consult
Norman Doidge, *The Brain That Changes Itself: Stories of Personal
Triumph from the Frontiers of Brain Science* (New York: Penguin, 2007).

Chapter 5: Working with Specific Pain Conditions

1. An excellent and comprehensive resource for further reading is
Wendy L. Cohan, RN, *The Better Bladder Book: A Holistic Approach
to Healing Interstitial Cystitis and Chronic Pelvic Pain* (New York:
Hunter House, 2010).

2. "Treating Interstitial Cystitis," *Harvard Medical School Family Health
Guide,* health.harvard.edu/fhg/updates/update0104d.shtml.

3. I. Castro et al., "Prevalence of Abuse in Fibromyalgia and Other Rheumatic
Disorders at a Specialized Clinic in Rheumatic Diseases in Guatemala
City," *Journal of Clinical Rheumatology* 11, No. 3 (June 2005): 140–45.

4. These two photos are from Peter Levine, *Healing Trauma:
A Pioneering Program for Restoring The Wisdom of Your Body* (Boulder,
CO: Sounds True, Pap/Com edition, 2008), 60.

5. The ventral vagal system is the social engagement, bonding, and relational function of the polyvagal system described by Dr. Stephen Porges, *The Polyvagal Theory: Neurophysiological Foundations of Emotions, Attachment, Communication, and Self-Regulation* (New York: W. W. Norton, 2011).

6. See the book/CD program by Tara Brach, *Radical Self-Acceptance: A Buddhist Guide to Freeing Yourself from Shame* (Boulder, CO: Sounds True, 2005). To order and hear a preview, go to soundstrue. com/shop/Radical-Self-Acceptance/330.productdetails.

7. This is one of the main protocols for clearing energy reversals. For more information and a diagram, see Maggie Phillips, *Reversing Chronic Pain,* 111–113.

8. For more information about the science of affirmations, please visit affirmativethinking.wordpress.com/science-of-affirmations-proof and hubpages.com/hub/self-affirmations.

9. To learn more about how to create new neuronal pathways, which is an application of neuroplasticity, visit whatisneuroplasticity.com/ pathways.php.

Chapter 6: Preventing and Resolving the Pain of Medical Trauma

1. You might also want to explore a very useful CD by Belleruth Naparstek called *Successful Surgery*, which we recommend highly. Other possibilities include audios recorded in consultation with a professional that are made especially for you.

2. Discussing the use of medications before, during, and after a medical procedure is highly important. For guidelines, please see mayoclinic. com/health/pain-medications/PN00060.

3. The Pain Patient Bill of Rights, created by the National Pain Foundation, can be found in its entirety at nationalpainfoundation. org/articles/295/patient-bill-of-rights.

4. For additional resources for effective ways of communicating with your doctor, including making decisions about who will perform

your surgery and whether or not you need surgery, visit
muschealth.com/safety/documents/choosingdr.pdf and poultry-line.
com/2010/03/how-to-decide-whether-to-have-surgery-or-not.html.

5. Please see healthpages.org/health-a-z/how-to-make-and-use-an-ice-
bag for information on how to make and use ice packs.

Chapter 7: Resilience, Continued Recovery, and Restoring the Deep Self

1. A more complete description of this process can be found in Levine,
In an Unspoken Voice, 73–95.

2. There is some evidence that Dr. Kabat-Zinn's Mindfulness-Based Stress
Reduction (MBSR) Program may increase left frontal lobe activity
resulting in greater ability to cope with stress. Please see Richard J.
Davidson, PhD, Jon Kabat-Zinn, PhD et al., "Alterations in Brain
and Immune Function Produced by Mindfulness Meditation,"
Psychosomatic Medicine 65 (2003): 564–70. You may also want
to read Dr. Kabat-Zinn's book *Full Catastrophe Living: Using the
Wisdom of Your Body and Mind to Face Stress, Pain, and Illness* (New
York: Delta, 1990) for a complete description of this program.

3. Intentions are very similar to affirmations. Although the distinction is murky, most people accept the difference that intentions are
global statements that encompass an overall attitude toward life (for
example, "I want to be a more compassionate person" or "I want
to learn how to support myself during the job interview process").
Affirmations are stated as if they are already happening (for example, "I am creating a happy relationship" or "I am living a happier
life"). Typically, these terms are used interchangeably; we believe
that it's important to use both. For more information on the effects
of affirmations, please refer to Sheila Bender and Mary Sise, *The
Energy of Belief: Psychology's Power Tools to Focus Intention and Release
Blocking Beliefs* (Fulton, CA: Energy Psychology Press, 2007). Also
see Belleruth Naparstek's excellent CD program, *Guided Imagery for*

the Three Stages of Healing Trauma: Nine Meditations for Posttraumatic Stress (Akron, OH: Health Journeys, 2005), which can be ordered at healthjourneys.com/Product_Detail.aspx?id=250.

4. For more information about the conflict-free deep self, see Maggie Phillips and Claire Frederick, *Empowering the Self Through Ego-State Therapy*, 2010, an ebook that can be ordered through reversingchronicpain.com

5. Peter Levine, *Healing Trauma*.

Suggested Reading
and Listening

Books by Peter A. Levine

Healing Trauma: A Pioneering Program for Restoring the Wisdom of Your Body. Boulder, CO: Sounds True, 2008.

In an Unspoken Voice: How the Body Releases Trauma and Restores Goodness. Berkeley, CA: North Atlantic Books, 2010.

Sexual Healing, Transforming the Sacred Wound (Audio CD). Boulder, CO: Sounds True, 2003.

Trauma-Proofing Your Kids; A Parent's Guide to Instilling Confidence, Joy and Resilience. Berkeley, CA: North Atlantic Books, 2009.

Waking the Tiger: Healing Trauma: The Innate Capacity to Transform Overwhelming Experiences. Berkeley, CA: North Atlantic Books, 1997.

Books by Maggie Phillips

Finding the Energy to Heal: How EMDR, Hypnosis, TFT, Imagery, and Body-Focused Therapy Can Help Restore Mindbody Health. New York: W. W. Norton, 2000.

Healing the Divided Self: Clinical and Ericksonian Hypnotherapy for Dissociative and Posttraumatic Conditions. New York: W. W. Norton, 1995.

Hypnosis: The Headache Solution (Audio CD). The Hypnosis Network, 2005.

Hypnosis: The Pain Solution (Audio CD). The Hypnosis Network, 2005.

Reversing Chronic Pain: A 10-Point All-Natural Plan for Lasting Relief. Berkeley, CA: North Atlantic Books, 2007.

Audios

Naparstek, Belleruth. *A Guided Meditation for Healing Trauma (PTSD).* Akron, OH: Health Journeys, 1999.

———. *A Meditation to Promote Successful Surgery.* Akron, OH: Health Journeys, 1992.

Rossman, Martin. *Preparing for Surgery: Guided Imagery Exercises for Relaxation and Accelerated Healing* (Audio CD). Boulder, CO: Sounds True, 2006.

See additional audio downloads with a variety of presenters, including Peter Levine, Kathy Kain, Marty Rossman, Laurel Parnell, and other experts at reversingchronicpain.com/products

Resources

Active Release Therapy

ART is one of the treatments of choice for soft tissue injuries resulting from overuse conditions, such as carpal tunnel syndrome. The technique involves shortening the tissue, applying careful contact to help stretch it in relation to adjacent tissues. ART training is comprehensive and the method has over 500 healing movements that are taught by certified trainers to qualified professionals, including chiropractors and physical therapists.

Acupoints

These are points on the body that are the focus of acupressure, acupuncture, and other Eastern or alternative medical treatments. Several hundred acupoints are located along the fourteen meridians, or energy pathways, first identified by the Chinese and believed to affect a specific organ or part of the body. These are approaches related to complementary and alternative medicine (CAM). Even though there is controversy about its efficacy, acupuncture has been accepted by the American Medical Association as an evidence-based treatment for pain and other conditions. This means acupuncture is considered integrative medicine, which is a blend of alternative approaches and conventional medicine. For more information, go to nccam.nih.gov/health/acupuncture.

Resources

Alexander Technique

An educational method designed to change movement habits. The technique is presented during a series of lessons that teach ease and freedom of movement, balance, and other skills that can be applied to sitting, walking, lying down, lifting, and other basic activities of everyday life. For more information, go to alexandertechnique.com/at.htm.

ASTYM

A rehabilitation method that helps to heal soft tissue, tendons, muscles, and ligaments by stimulating regeneration. It is noninvasive and recommended for treating plantar fasciitis, scar tissue, and various types of body pain, such as Achilles tendon tears. Research studies and other information can be found at astym.com/professionals/research.asp.

Body Scan

A step-by-step tour of your body, which may begin as you notice points of contact with the mat or floor underneath you if you are lying down or sitting. Usually the tour begins with one of your feet, and continues systematically to the other foot, calves, legs, and so on, to the top of your head. Your general intention is to stay present in the current moment throughout and then to connect with the entire body. The purpose is to bring your awareness to each part of your body sequentially, not to try to change your body experience but to notice and accept what's there, although there is a softening and a letting go that can happen as you scan. For more information, see meditation-techniques-for-happiness.com/body-scan-meditation.html.

EMDR (Eye Movement Desensitization and Reprocessing)

This method was developed by research psychologist Dr. Francine Shapiro to help resolve trauma-related difficulties. Originally used with such problems as rape and combat trauma, EMDR is now used with many other symptoms, including chronic pain and stress. According to Shapiro's theory, trauma overwhelms neurological and cognitive processing networks, and the goal of EMDR is to assist in reprocessing so that elements of trauma lose their negative charge. EMDR uses an eight-step model to address various aspects of previous experience that have been traumatizing or distressing. Bilateral stimulation through lateral eye movements, tapping on the knees or hands, or bilateral audio tones are used while the client is focused on distressing elements of past experience. More recently, EMDR has been used to develop resources prior to trauma processing. We strongly recommend, especially if you have significant trauma in your history, that if you use EMDR, you work with an EMDR therapist who is skilled with resource installation as well as trauma processing. For more information on EMDR and help finding a qualified practitioner, please go to emdr.com.

Energy Approaches

Many energy approaches can be helpful with pain and have the benefit of very rarely creating negative effects. These include EFT (emotional freedom techniques), TFT (thought field therapy), EDxTm (energy diagnostic and treatment methods), WHEE (Whole Health-Easily and Effectively®), and reiki, acupuncture, and qi gong. For more information on these and other energy approaches, go to energypsych.org, or see Maggie Phillips, *Reversing Chronic Pain,* and David Feinstein, Donna Eden, and Gary Craig, *The Promise of Energy Psychology: Revolutionary Tool for Dramatic Personal Change* (New York: Tarcher, 2005). Generally, the evidence for these methods is anecdotal case studies, though more scientific studies are underway.

In chapter 2 (page 19), we include the over-energy correction (Cook's Hookup), which is especially useful with symptoms related to anxiety and panic. Here are the steps for this valuable tool derived from applied kinesiology:

1. Cross your left ankle over right.
2. Extend both arms in front of you, hands back to back.
3. Cross right hand over left at wrist and clasp fingers together, interlocked.
4. Roll and tuck clasped hands toward you, and rest them comfortably on your chest.
5. Inhale slowly through nose, tongue up in mouth. Exhale through mouth, tongue down.
6. Hold this pose, gently, and continue slow, deep breathing for one to two minutes.

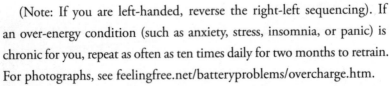

(Note: If you are left-handed, reverse the right-left sequencing). If an over-energy condition (such as anxiety, stress, insomnia, or panic) is chronic for you, repeat as often as ten times daily for two months to retrain. For photographs, see feelingfree.net/batteryproblems/overcharge.htm.

In chapter 5 (page 82), we include the concept of psychological reversal, a barrier to energy flow, which consists of one flow in the direction of positive intention for change opposed by another flow of energy away from change. For additional methods beyond the one that involves rubbing the "sore spots" on the chest an inch below the collarbone and four to five inches toward the shoulder crease, see energycoachonline.com/?p=21.

Feldenkrais Method

A method of somatic education and integration. Awareness through movement is taught through practice exercises presented to groups. These lessons attempt to make you aware of habitual neuromuscular patterns and rigidities, and to expand options for new ways of moving while increasing sensitivity and improving efficiency. Functional integration lessons are used with individuals to guide them through movements with gentle, noninvasive touching. For more information, see feldenkrais.com.

Journaling

A learning tool that has gained popularity and evidence of success over the last twenty years. Ira Progoff was one of the first professionals to see the value of intensive journaling for personal growth and development. In its various forms, journaling can help you become aware of and record your thoughts, daily experiences, and evolving insights. We have found that structured assignments are most helpful with people who have pain and have included these throughout the Freedom from Pain program. These assignments invite you to journal about your experiences with the fourteen audio exercises, helping you to note shifts in daily pain patterns as you practice the skills and principles we present. For more information about the uses and benefits of journaling, type "evidence for journaling" in your Internet search engine for a listing of numerous articles.

Laser Therapy

Used as a medical treatment with many types of pain. Low-level laser therapy (LLLT) is often administered via "cold lasers" and varies the intensity and location of light waves. Specific protocols for LLLT have demonstrated effectiveness with rheumatoid arthritis, osteoarthritis, acute and chronic neck pain, and tendonitis. It is more controversial in its uses with back pain, dentistry, and wound healing. Higher intensity laser therapy is also used to cut, burn, or remove tissue as a form of noninvasive therapy. See blue.regence.com/trgmedpol/medicine/med105.html.

Massage/Self-Massage

A body therapy that manipulates muscle and connective tissue to relieve pain, promote relaxation, enhance healing, and promote better mobility usually using pressure applied by the hands, elbows, forearms, fingers (in some cases also the knees and feet) of the practitioner. Massage may also entail work with tendons, ligaments, the lymphatic system, and gastrointestinal system. According to Wikipedia alone, there are over eighty kinds of recognized massage. These include shiatsu, deep tissue, Swedish, polarity, and Thai massage.

Mindfulness Practices

Dr. Jon Kabat-Zinn is the creator of mindfulness-based stress reduction (MBSR) programs developed at Harvard Medical School and now implemented in many hospitals and clinics worldwide. To access video and audio presentations by Dr. Kabat-Zinn, visit mindfulnesstapes.com and youtube.com/watch?v=3nwwKbM_vJc.

Movement

Many types of movement techniques can be used to enhance recovery from pain. Examples are yoga, qi gong, tai chi, and stretching. Dance and movement therapy is the therapeutic use of dance and movement to promote integration at social, cognitive, emotional, physical, and social levels. For more information, see adta.org.

Nutritional Supplements

These have become increasingly popular in recent years and include vitamins, minerals, herbs or botanicals, amino acids, and homeopathic remedies that may help relieve many types of pain, including nerve pain, and related inflammation. The Food and Drug Administration regulates these substances as a type of food rather than drug. For more information, use Google to explore specific supplements of interest or visit everydayhealth.com/pain-management/6-food-additives-to-subtract-from-your-diet.aspx.

Pilates

A physical fitness/rehabilitation system developed by Joseph Pilates, pilates teaches a series of protocols designed to increase strength, flexibility, and control of the body. Although originally used to help dancers to recover from injuries, Pilates is now used for general conditioning and fitness. To read more and find a Pilates teacher, visit medicinenet.com/pilates/article.htm.

Radical Self-Acceptance

A type of meditation program based on Buddhist principles and mindfulness practice designed to help free you from shame. Tara Brach is one of the experts on this approach and has developed a book/CD program called *Radical Self-Acceptance: A Buddhist Guide to Freeing Yourself from Shame* (Sounds True, 2005) and has also published *Radical Acceptance: Embracing Your Life with the Heart of a Buddha* (New York: Bantam, 2004).

Self-Hypnosis

The process of guiding yourself into a pleasant, voluntary state of relaxed attention during which the conscious critical mind is more relaxed and the subconscious critical mind is more active in a self-regulated manner. The benefits of self-hypnosis center on its initiation and promotion of positive self-change. You can learn self-hypnosis from a good book, audio program, and/or skilled and experienced professional. We recommend *Hypnosis: The Pain Solution,* a CD program by Maggie Phillips that teaches self-hypnosis for the regulation of pain and discomfort (hypnosisnetwork.com/hypnosis/pain_management.php), and the book by Bruce Eimer, *Hypnotize Yourself Out of Pain Now!* (hypnosis helpcenter.net/hypnosis/book.html).

Somatic Experiencing

A body-awareness approach to trauma developed by Peter A. Levine from over forty years of study, research, and hands-on development. The method is based on the principle that human beings, like other animals, have an innate capacity to overcome and transform many effects of trauma. For additional information, please see traumahealing.com and somaticexperiencing.com.

TENS Units

TENS (transcutaneous electrical nerve stimulation) devices have been particularly useful for various types of nerve pain. They stimulate nerves through electrodes attached to the skin. A typical battery-operated TENS unit modulates pulse width, frequency, and intensity of pain and so is very helpful in self-regulation. TENS units can help to shift the sensations of pain by introducing a competing sensation that can be fully regulated by the pain patient. Please visit wikipedia.org/wiki/Transcutaneous_electrical_nerve_stimulation for more information.

Index

Index

B

back pain, 86–92

barriers to recovery, resolving, 79–81

beliefs, 24, 46

brain/body chemistry and, 113

negative beliefs/myths, 54–57, 79–81

"Bill of Rights" for pain patients, 134, 159n3

blood clotting, nutritional supplements and, 137

body. *See also* sensation
    as ally/friend, 6, 16–17, 140
    awareness skills, 57–71, 140
    disconnection/dissociation from, 6, 28
    embodied awareness, 57–59, 65–66, 140
    healing through, 6, 140
    movement practices, 7–8
    physical pain and, 3
    re-inhabiting (exercise), 8–9
    reconnecting with, 8–9, 29, 32–33
    resting place in (exercise), 31–32, 38
    sensation and, 6–9

body scan, 30, 154n1, 166

body sensations. *See* sensation

body tapping, 60

Bonheim, Jalaja, 139

bracing reactions, 19, 20, 40, 89, 93
    working with, 89–92

brain, 19, 23–24

brain scans, 23–24

brain stem, 111–118
    cortex, 23–24, 65
    mindfulness and, 65–66
    plasticity, 78, 112–113, 158n12

breakthrough pain, 57

breathing, 33–36, 124–125
    ahh sound, 125
    circle breathing, 24–26, 36, 64, 154n2
    controlled, 35
    depression and, 108
    diaphragmatic breathing, 34–35, 63–64
    exhalation, focus on, 34–35

heart and, 75

Just One Breath exercise, 33–34, 125

positive regulation of, 35–36

pre-surgical exercises, 124–125

re-inhabiting the body exercise, 8–9

for shifting dissociation, 33–36, 63–64

sounds with, 124–125

voo breathing, 34–35, 125

Buddha, 1

burning sensations, 104

C

cerebral cortex, 24

charge, discharge, and settle responses, 14–16

childhood trauma, xiii, 85

chronic depression, 106–115

chronic fatigue, 92

chronic pain, 27–52
    neck, back, and shoulder pain, 86–92
    preventing, 2
    shift from normal pain to, 27–28
    techniques for neutralizing, 27–52
    trauma and, xi–xiii, 22–23, 86
    working with medical professionals on, 54

chronic regional pain syndrome (CRPS), 104–105

circle breathing, 24–26, 36, 64, 154n2

clotting, nutritional supplements and, 137

cognitive therapies, 147–148

collapsed posture, 41–42

compassion, 75–77, 148

conflict-free experience, 42–43, 156n8

connection, 64–65

contraction, 1, 19, 68–69

Cook's Hookup, 43, 156n9, 167

cortex (of brain), 23–24, 65

cortisol, 37–38, 155n4

CRPS (chronic regional pain syndrome), 104–106

Index

charge, discharge, and settle
responses, 14–16
childhood, xiii, 85
chronic pain and, xi-xiii, 22–23,
27, 86
cumulative trauma disorder,
136–137
developmental, 85
dissociation or freezing and, 69
fear and, 28
levels of, 84–86
medical trauma, pain of, 117–138
memory and, 37, 154–155n3
pain and, 6, 22–23, 84–86
past, current pain related to, 22–23,
84–85
past, minimizing impact of,
128–131
precipitating events, xii
reactions to, 27–52
recovery from. *See* recovery;
resilience
repeated/repetitive, 5, 136–137
single vs. multiple-ongoing events,
5, 85
surgical. *See* medical trauma/
medical procedures
techniques for addressing, xii-xiii,
27–52
threat response and, 12–14
unresolved, effect on pain, xi-xiii,
22–23, 37, 84–86
unresolved, releasing, 23
wild animals and, 5, 14–16

Trauma Spectrum, The (Scaer), 41
triggers, interrupting, 67–68
triumph, 143–144

U

ultrasound, 136
unmanageable pain, strategies for,
53–82
Unspoken Voice, In an (Levine), 58

V

vagus, 109
ventral vagal system, 109, 148, 159n5
voo breathing, 34–35, 125

W

walk around the block, 106–107
WHEE (Whole Health-Easily and
Effectively), 167
wholeness, xv, xx, 52, 71–72, 140, 150
wild animals, 5, 14–16

Y

yoga, xi, 7

About the Authors

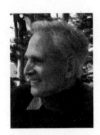**Peter A. Levine, PhD,** holds doctorates in medical bio-physics and psychology. He is the developer of Somatic Experiencing®, a body-based, naturalistic approach to healing trauma, which he has developed during the past forty years. He has received the Lifetime Achievement Award from the United States Association for Body Psychotherapy (USABP), in recognition of his original and pioneering work in trauma. He also received an honorary award as the Reiss-Davis Chair for his lifetime contributions to infant and child psychiatry.

Dr. Levine served as a stress consultant for NASA in the early space shuttle development. He has served on the APA (American Psychological Association) President's Initiative and the International Psychologists for Social Responsibility Task Force for responding to large-scale disasters and ethno-political warfare.

He is the author of several bestselling books on trauma, including *Waking the Tiger, Healing Trauma,* published in twenty-four languages, *Trauma Through a Child's Eyes,* and *Trauma-Proofing Your Kids: A Parent's Guide for Instilling Confidence, Joy and Resilience.* His most recent ("magnum opus") book is *In an Unspoken Voice: How the Body Releases Trauma and Restores Goodness.* More information is available at traumahealing.com and somaticexperiencing.com.

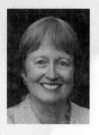

Maggie Phillips, PhD, lives and works as a licensed clinical psychologist in Oakland Hills above San Francisco Bay. As the author of three previous books and numerous papers, chapters, and articles on trauma, dissociation, pain, ego-state therapy, hypnosis, and mind-body healing, she specializes in the treatment of traumatic stress, dissociative, and pain disorders. She is a fellow of the American Society of Clinical Hypnosis and corecipient of its Crasilneck award for the best writing in the field of hypnosis. She is also a fellow of the International Society for the Study of Trauma and Dissociation, and corecipient of its Cornelia Wilbur award for her contributions to the treatment of dissociation. She has taught at major conferences and presented invited workshops on Somatic Experiencing, trauma, hypnosis, Ego-State Therapy, EMDR, behavioral medicine, and Energy Psychology in the US, the UK, Canada, Europe, South Africa, Australia, Scandinavia, Hong Kong, China, Malaysia, and Japan. Her most recent, best-selling book, *Reversing Chronic Pain: A 10-Point All-Natural Plan for Lasting Relief,* was released by North Atlantic Books in October 2007.

Dr. Phillips is the creator of a companion online pain self-help program and a pain CD coaching program available at reversingchronicpain.com. She is also the creator and host of a popular monthly teleseminar and newsletter series (maggiephillipsphd.com), which have featured several e-courses copresented with Peter Levine, including an audio series on somatic approaches to treating pain and trauma, which provided the genesis for their current joint book, *Freedom from Pain.* She has also recorded two pain CD programs, *Hypnosis: The Pain Solution* and *Hypnosis: The Headache Solution,* distributed by hypnosisnetwork.com. Her other books are *Finding the Energy to Heal* (W. W. Norton, 2000) and *Healing the Divided Self* (W. W. Norton, 1995), co-authored with Dr. Claire Frederick, MD. As an innovator in mind-body healing and in the treatment of persistent pain and trauma, Dr. Phillips is particularly interested in the interface of trauma, dissociation, and emotional and physical pain conditions.

About Sounds True

SOUNDS TRUE IS A MULTIMEDIA PUBLISHER whose mission is to inspire and support personal transformation and spiritual awakening. Founded in 1985 and located in Boulder, Colorado, we work with many of the leading spiritual teachers, thinkers, healers, and visionary artists of our time. We strive with every title to preserve the essential "living wisdom" of the author or artist. It is our goal to create products that not only provide information to a reader or listener, but that also embody the quality of a wisdom transmission.

For those seeking genuine transformation, Sounds True is your trusted partner. At SoundsTrue.com you will find a wealth of free resources to support your journey, including exclusive weekly audio interviews, free downloads, interactive learning tools, and other special savings on all our titles.

To listen to a podcast interview with Sounds True publisher Tami Simon and authors Peter Levine and Maggie Phillips, visit SoundsTrue.com/bonus/LevineFreedom.

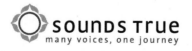

SOUNDS TRUE
many voices, one journey